Women and Smoking
in America, 1880–1950

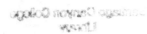

ALSO BY KERRY SEGRAVE
AND FROM MCFARLAND

Endorsements in Advertising: A Social History (2005)

Foreign Films in America: A History (2004)

Lie Detectors: A Social History (2004)

Product Placement in Hollywood Films: A History (2004)

Piracy in the Motion Picture Industry (2003)

Jukeboxes: An American Social History (2002)

Vending Machines: An American Social History (2002)

Age Discrimination by Employers (2001)

Shoplifting: A Social History (2001)

Movies at Home: How Hollywood Came to Television (1999)

*American Television Abroad: Hollywood's Attempt to
Dominate World Television* (1998)

Tipping: An American Social History of Gratuities (1998)

*American Films Abroad: Hollywood's Domination of
the World's Movie Screens from the 1890s to the Present* (1997)

Baldness: A Social History (1996)

Policewomen: A History (1995)

Payola in the Music Industry: A History, 1880–1991 (1994)

*The Sexual Harassment of Women
in the Workplace, 1600 to 1993* (1994)

Drive-in Theaters: A History from Their Inception in 1933 (1992)

*Women Serial and Mass Murderers: A Worldwide Reference,
1580 through 1990* (1992)

BY KERRY SEGRAVE AND LINDA MARTIN
AND FROM MCFARLAND

*The Continental Actress: European Film Stars of the Postwar Era;
Biographies, Criticism, Filmographies, Bibliographies* (1990)

*The Post Feminist Hollywood Actress: Biographies and
Filmographies of Stars Born After 1939* (1990)

Women and Smoking in America, 1880–1950

KERRY SEGRAVE

McFarland & Company, Inc., Publishers
OCM 60835251
Jefferson, North Carolina, and London

Library of Congress Online Catalog

Segrave, Kerry, 1944–
    Women and smoking in America, 1880–1950 / Kerry Segrave.
    p.   cm.
    Includes bibliographical references and index.

    ISBN 0-7864-2212-2 (softcover : 50# alkaline paper) ∞

    1. Women — Tobacco use — United States — History.
  2. Women — United States — Social conditions — 19th century.
  3. Women — United States — Social conditions — 20th century.
  I. Title.
  HV5746+   2005016991

British Library cataloguing data are available

Cover photograph: Carole Lombard in a publicity pose, about 1934

Manufactured in the United States of America

McFarland & Company, Inc., Publishers
  Box 611, Jefferson, North Carolina 28640
    www.mcfarlandpub.com

Contents

Preface

This book looks at women and smoking in America from 1880 to 1950. It was a period of time that could be described as the innocent years. Of course, there were accurate medical warnings about the dangers of smoking throughout this period, but they were ignored. In this timeframe the cigarette moved from being a maligned form of tobacco consumption, compared to cigars and pipes, to being the favored form of tobacco consumption by men and, really, the only form of tobacco used by women. By 1950 the cigarette smoker and smoking were widely accepted as part of America's social fabric, a social and companionable thing to do, a habit indulged in by men and women. By 1950 women smokers enjoyed the same degree of acceptance as did male smokers. How that came about is the subject of this book, as is the opposition to smoking in general by women.

The years divide neatly into four periods. In the first phase, from 1880 to 1908, the topic became subject to both media and public attention for the first time. Smoking by women did not take place in any public places; no restaurants permitted it, for example. Men, of course, smoked anywhere and everywhere, but mostly not cigarettes. According to accounts, what smoking that did take place was limited mainly to upper-class women who smoked covertly, at home, at private parties, and at socials—gatherings held by the upper class and for the upper class. Opposition was strong and based mostly on supposed moral transgressions committed by women who indulged.

During the period 1908–1919, women smokers went public in greater numbers and challenged the prejudices against smoking that applied to them alone. No restaurants in America officially permitted women to smoke at the start of this period, but most did by 1919. Mainly that was due to pressure placed on the establishments by women. Still, there was little smoking by women in other public places. Smoking in the street could and did land a number of women in jail.

More gains were made by female smokers in the period 1919–1927 when the practice took hold in American colleges. Almost no American institution of higher learning allowed women to smoke anywhere within its jurisdiction (and often out of it) in 1920; by around 1925–1926, most did, although conditions were often imposed. Smoking by women had come a long way by 1927 and it had all taken place without any cigarette advertising aimed directly at females.

Over the final period, 1927–1950, that deficiency was addressed as advertisers targeted women more. By 1927 it had become safe for advertisers to do so. Opposition movements had faded away, and the last of the laws that barred adults from buying cigarettes (none were enforced to any degree) was repealed.

After a long struggle, women smokers had gained full equality with make smokers by 1950. Most men then smoked, and at least one-third of women indulged. Most people felt it to be a sociable and harmless practice. Then, at the start of the 1950s, the health warnings increased and were more forceful, and attention began to be paid to them. The innocent years were over.

Research for this book was conducted at the University of British Columbia, Simon Fraser University, and the Vancouver Public Library, using various online and traditional databases.

1

The Years to 1880

"When I had taken two or three pipes, I was presently ready for another."
— Mary Rowlandson, 1670s

"When one hears of sly cigarettes between feminine lips at croquet parties, there is no more to be said."
— Mortimer Collins, 1869

The consumption of tobacco by women began to draw serious attention around 1880; however, their association with it went back at least to the 1600s. According to Alfred Dunhill, writing in 1925, in England in the 17th century the smoking of a clay pipe was well established among women in most classes of society. He thought it unsurprising to find a woodcut from that period of the famous Moll Cutpurse, a highway robber and generally bad character, puffing away on a pipe. But in another class of society, even Quaker ladies were said to have smoked pipes. One supposed impetus to the spread of the pipe-smoking habit among females was the reputed disinfectant value of tobacco against the plague. Such a belief was then fairly common among men and women. A French visitor to England in 1672 remarked that English women even provided their children with pipes—for their purported medicinal value. Around 1699 another French visitor reported the pipe to be in constant use by men and women. Within France, the daughters of Louis XIV were said to have been discovered one day by their brother, the Dauphin, smoking pipes lent to them by Swiss Guard officers. Louis XIV was averse to tobacco. As early as the 17th century, women in India and Africa were said to be heavy pipe smokers. By the time his account was published, Dunhill declared that females in the Western world had been induced by the cigarette to abandon the pipe. While he thought that a few remained faithful to the pipe, they indulged in the habit in private. "Those who venture to smoke a pipe in public are extremely few ... and do so in a spirit of bravado," stated Dunhill.[1]

In his book on the history of smoking, published in England in 1914, G. L. Apperson noted that although there existed some references to smoking by women that dated prior to the early 1600s, none of them could be confirmed, and they may not have been factual. On the other hand, he noted, "It is certain that from comparatively early in the seventeenth century there were to be found here and there women who smoked." He also mentioned Cutpurse and that on the title page of Thomas Middleton's comedy *The Roaring Girle* (1611), appeared a picture of the heroine, dressed in man's apparel and smoking a pipe from which issued a large cloud of smoke. In the course of the trial from an early libel action brought in the court of the archdeacon of Essex, it was disclosed that George Thresher sold beer and tobacco at his shop and that a good friend and customer of his was Elizabeth Savage, who came to his store many times to buy tobacco for herself. Apperson also noted that women tobacco smokers were not confined to any one class of society. The Reverend Giles Moore, rector of Horsted Keynes, Sussex, made a note in his journal and account book in 1665 of "Tobacco for my wife, 3d." In a letter from 1652 or 1653, Susan Crane wrote to her husband (then away on business), telling him she had used up all the tobacco he had left her and would he please send her some more — soon. Edmond Howes, who edited Stow's *Chronicles*, declared in 1631 that tobacco was "at this day commonly used by most men and many women."[2]

Still, Apperson felt that anything like general smoking by women in 17th century England appeared to have been confined to certain parts of the country, such as the west of England. From the evidence found he believed it was fair to conclude that during the 17th century smoking was not fashionable, or anything but rare, "among the women of the more well-to-do classes, while among women of humbler rank it was an occasional, and in a few districts a fairly general habit. The same conclusion holds good for the eighteenth century. Among women of the lowest class smoking was probably common enough." In Henry Fielding's *Amelia*, a woman of the "lowest character" was spoken of as smoking tobacco, drinking punch, talking obscenely and swearing and cursing — none of which were hallmarks of respectable females. A list of the provisions put on board the ship in which certain Quakers — Samuel Fothergill, Mary Peisly, Katherine Payton, and others — sailed on from Philadelphia to England in June 1756 indicated the women's storage chest contained, among other items, tobacco.[3]

With respect to Victorian England days, Apperson observed that there had always been pipe smokers among the women of the poorer classes with smoking being very common among the hard-working women of Northumberland and the Scottish border, up to the middle of the 1800s. In 1856 the *Darlington and Stockton Times* recorded the death on December 10, at Wallbury, Yorkshire, of Jane Garbutt, supposedly age 110. She retained all of her faculties up to her death and enjoyed her pipe to the end. A year before she died she was asked how long she had smoked: "Very nigh a hundred years," she replied. Pheasy Molly, for years an "inveterate smoker," died at Buxton in 1845, aged a reported 96. Her death was caused by the accidental ignition of her clothes as she was lighting her pipe at the fire. More than once in the past she had burned herself while engaged in the same task. Elderly Irish women, who were once a familiar feature of London street life as sellers of apples and other small items at street corners during this period, were often hardened smokers. Up to about the middle of Queen Victoria's reign (she ruled from 1837–1901) female smoking in 19th century England was pretty much confined, said Apperson, to the lower classes. Respectable people in the middle and upper classes, he declared, would have been horrified at the idea of a pipe or a cigar between feminine lips; cigarettes had been used by men for a long time before it began to be whispered that here and there a lady — "who was usually considered dreadfully 'fast' for her pains" — indulged in a cigarette. He said it was in the 1860s that cigarette smoking by women began to creep in. Mortimer Collins, writing in 1869 in a piece against the use of tobacco by young men, added in a shocked digression: "When one hears of sly cigarettes between feminine lips at croquet parties, there is no more to be said."[4]

Arguing that smoking by women was indeed rare in Victorian England, a correspondent in the *Times* of London in 1926 said flatly there was no evidence that women smoked in Victorian days. According to this source John Leech, whose drawings and sketches of all classes of society covered a couple of decades in this period, never depicted even the "fastest" of his young women as indulging in tobacco. Nor did that depicter of manners at home and abroad, William M. Thackeray (1811–1863) ever allude to such a habit as being prevalent or even existent among women. Finally, going back even further, argued the correspondent, one could search the pages of the *Spectator* in vain for any mention of that kind of indulgence among the many forms of female foibles censured therein over time. As far as this correspondent was concerned the practice of women smoking "took on" from the time when King Edward VII (1844–1910, reigned from 1901–1910), as Prince of Wales (he assumed that title as an infant), initiated the custom of smoking at the dinner table and that it made its way by degrees through all grades of society.[5]

That article prompted a number of replies in the form of letters to the editor. One said there was a reference in Thackeray's works to women smoking, citing *Pendennis* (1848–1850) volume 2, chapter 3. Admittedly the letter writer knew of no other such references in Thackeray's works. Another person wrote to say that in *Punch* of August 29, 1857, a drawing by Leech featured a young lady taking a cigar from her case. In response to that, still another writer declared that in that drawing Leech was only kidding; he was portraying impossibilities or visions, not reality. Leech had a series of verses called "Surprises," also, and the vignette to those verses showed a woman smoking a cigarette.[6]

Over in America, Cassandra Tate, in her history of smoking, said that records of colonist court proceedings in New England included numerous casual references to women smoking, with nothing to indicate that the practice was out of the ordinary. Testimony in several rape trials was said to indicate that it was acceptable for women to smoke at their own hearths or doorsteps but not in taverns, especially in the company of strangers. In rural areas, midwives often prescribed an analgesic pipe for women in labor. Mary Rowlandson, pious wife of a Puritan minister, came to regret her use of tobacco and gave it up after being captured by Indians in Massachusetts in 1676. During her addiction to the weed, she said, "When I had taken two or three pipes, I was presently ready for another." Benjamin Ferris, a Quaker traveling in western New York around 1825 was upset to find women so "infected by the tobacco plague" that "they sit smoking their pipes by the half dozen without the least attempt to conceal it, or the least apparent sense of its indelicacy." Such smoking women may have been even more common in the South. Durand de Dauphine, a French Huguenot traveling in Virginia and Maryland in 1686, observed women smoking "everywhere," even in church. Anecdotal evidence was said to suggest that Southern women continued using pipes long after their Northern counterparts gave them up. Tobacco use was reported to have been found at all levels of female society in the antebellum South, from the backwoods to the White House. The wives of presidents Andrew Jackson (1829–1837) and Zachary Taylor (1849–1850) were said to both be ardent pipe smokers, while Dolley Madison (her husband James Madison was president from 1809 to 1817) also indulged in an occasional pipe although she preferred snuff (powered tobacco) and often used it publicly during her tenure as first lady. A Wyoming pioneer by the name of W. S. Kimball vividly recalled "many good women" who smoked corncob or clay pipes in his native Kentucky during the Civil War era.[7]

An article that appeared in the New York Times in 1894 remarked that a half century earlier, around 1844, in Connecticut "many gentlewomen smoked with delight — not the graceful cigarette of to-day, but pipes!"[8]

By the late 1870s or so, the habit of American women smoking cigarettes was for the most part considered the province of chorus girls, actresses, prostitutes and other women of doubtful reputation, wrote Tate. As the New York Times said in 1879: "The practice of cigarette-smoking among ladies seems to be generally regarded as the usual accompaniment of, or prelude to, immorality." One of the earliest extant photographs of anyone with a cigarette, taken around 1850, featured Irish entertainer Lola Montez, shown with a cigarette between her fingers. Victorian actress Lillie Langtry (mistress of Britain's future King Edward VII) scandalized society by posing with a cigarette in her mouth. Georges Bizet's opera Carmen (produced in New York for the first time in 1878 and popular with American audiences through the 1880s and 1890s) helped strengthen the link between women, cigarettes and sin. Bizet's heroine, who worked in a cigarette factory in Spain and regularly smoked the product she helped manufacture, was vulgar and sensual — qualities that were regularly ascribed to female smokers for some time to come. So unsettling was this connection that in a production of Carmen on the Chautauqua circuit in Kansas in 1914, the story was changed so that the heroine worked in a dairy instead of a cigarette factory. She made her entrance carrying a milk pail instead of a smoke.[9]

According to a 1906 report, people then upset by women smoking would have been worse off around 1846 because they would have seen five times as many women taking snuff as were then indulging in cigarettes. That old habit, "after standing undismayed in reputable society for many a decade, went into a decline half a century ago [1856] and is now almost extinct." If the cigarette was equally as unwholesome as was snuff, the reporter thought, it was "certainly less offensive to the refined taste."[10]

Despite that account, an 1874 piece declared there were increasing numbers of women taking snuff in all parts of the United States, especially in the South. But the increase was not surprising to the reporter, "when we consider the large increase of nervous excitement to which the women of the day are exposed in comparison with the placid course of the lives of their grandmothers fifty years ago." A favored method for women taking snuff was by dipping. The user (or dipper) was provided with a small spoon, around half the size of a common teaspoon, with which she dipped a sufficient quantity of snuff from her bottle. Then seizing her lower lip with the thumb and forefinger of her left hand, she drew it well forward and filled the cavity with the snuff contained in the spoon. There she let it remain until it was gradually diffused through her mouth, expectorating all the while "in a manner that would do credit to a veteran." Snuff was said to be popular especially with factory girls in all the eastern states.[11]

Visiting a well-known jeweler in New York City in 1899, a reporter for the *Sun* newspaper discovered that this store — which sold various smoking "necessities" to women — still sold a lot of snuff to women. Most of that business was transacted by mail or by maid; few of the women who used snuff actually came into his store to buy their supply directly.[12]

By the end of the 1870s, it appeared that smoking among women in America or elsewhere was a fairly unusual occurrence. To the extent that it took place at all it was spread through all of society's classes, perhaps more so in the lower classes. Tobacco consumption by women was more likely to be through the pipe, or even snuff, than through the cigarette, but all that changed by the end of the 1870s as smoking by women came to focus almost exclusively on the cigarette. Over time the odd article appeared talking abut women turning to pipes (usually in response to some threatened shortage of tobacco during war time) or, more rarely, even cigars, but for all intents and purposes the link joining women and smoking would always be the cigarette. Already by the 1870s a link between women smoking cigarettes and immorality had been established. Partly that was due to the use of cigarettes by show business women — people with more uninhibited lifestyles and less under the restraint of social convention. Partly, it was because the cigarette did not start off by being accepted with open arms. Its status and reputation were poor to start with.

2

The Status of the Cigarette, 1860s–1930s

"You ask me what we need to win this war. I answer tobacco as much as bullets."
— General John J. Pershing, during World War I

Around 1869, according to journalist Eunice Fuller Barnard, fewer cigarettes were smoked in America in a single year than were consumed in a single day in 1929. Not only were reformers and lawmakers against them in the late 1800s, but so was American general opinion. No real man, it was assumed, would lower himself to touch them. For some obscure reason they were thought to be more effeminate and more vicious than any other form of tobacco. Cigarettes got going in the United States in the 1870s, said Barnard (20 to 30 years earlier in Europe), with the advent of new production methods that decade that allowed them to be retailed at 10 for a nickel. Real men in America smoked cigars, and pipes to a much lesser degree, but the newer and cheaper price made cigarettes more attractive. In the 1880s, explained Barnard, banks and offices prohibited cigarette smoking but allowed cigar puffing (to men only, of course). Critics declared the cigarette to be a "thing of evil." Rumors circulated that cigarettes were doped with substances, such as opium, and the paper wrappers around the tobacco also contained dangerous substances, such as arsenic. So persistent were such rumors that various state and university laboratories went so far as to run tests disproving those allegations, as did the U.S. Department of Agriculture, but the stories stubbornly circulated for years. At best, a cigarette in place of a cigar or pipe was looked on by the majority of people as a debasement of manhood. By 1899 or so the despised "coffin nails" were not only rejected by men but also banned by

9

law in some states. By around 1897, for the first time, as many cigarettes were consumed in the United States as cigars. It was not until 1910 that they at last came to permanently exceed the cigar in use, as they declined somewhat after 1897 due to the pressure placed on them by reformers. A rehabilitation of the cigarette did not take place completely until World War I. During that conflict the YMCA lifted its ban on smoking and sent 70 million cigarettes overseas to U.S. forces. Other relief and social organizations did the same thing, and smokes for American fighting forces became a popular form of war contribution. Thus the cigarette gained a respectable foothold in America by the end of World War I.[1]

With the entry of the United States into World War I, the cigarette opposition became considerably blunted as generals and commanders of the troops were more concerned with sobriety and chastity than tobacco and, reportedly, actually encouraged its use in the effective absence of alcohol and women. Apparently, the underpinnings of the theory held that one could not take all the vices away from troops without running the risk of serious dysfunction. Supplying tobacco was seen as the vice that was easiest to cater to while not impairing troop efficiency. "Smokes for soldiers" was a civilian campaign started in June 1917 that distributed thousands of cigarettes in the short time the United States was involved in the war. Newspapers all over America displayed headlines and advertising leads such as, "Our Army in France Is Short of Tobacco," "Boys at Front Need Tobacco," and "I Need Smokes More Than Anything Else."[2]

Consumption of cigarettes (in millions) in America was as follows, by decade; 1870, 13.9 cigarettes, 0.36 per capita consumption; 1880, 408.7, 8.19; 1890, 2,233.3, 35.48; 1900, 2,635.4, 34.68; 1910, 7,862.3, 85.49; 1920, 50,408.8, 470.85; 1930, 119,941.3, 976.91. One could see from the numbers the dramatic increase in cigarette consumption between 1910 and 1920, much of it due to the influence of the war, an increase that continued from 1920 to 1930. By 1890, 26 states had enacted laws prohibiting the sale of cigarettes to minors, but much to their disappointment, members of the anticigarette movement, who had been responsible for those laws being placed on the books, found those laws did not stop smoking among youth. By the end of 1909, Arkansas, Illinois, Indiana, Iowa, Kansas, Michigan, Minnesota, Missouri, Nebraska, New Hampshire, North Dakota, Oklahoma, South Dakota, Washington and Wisconsin had enacted statutes totally prohibiting the sale of cigarettes (to all people); Tennessee and West Virginia imposed such heavy taxes on cigarettes that the effect was the same as prohibition. Despite those legal barriers (enforcement of all those statutes was close to nil) cigarette consumption kept increasing. That increase continued despite the fact that popular attitudes were also anticigarette, explained authors Ronald Troyer and Gerald Markle. Among women, cigarette smoking was seen as a symbol of the prostitute, while men's use was viewed as effeminate. Clearly, the cigarette did not represent propriety and sophistication.[3]

Troyer and Markle added that World War I rehabilitated the cigarette as its supply to the forces overseas was quickly elevated to being a vital part of the war effort. General John J. Pershing was reported to have cabled Washington, D.C.: "Tobacco is as indispensable as the daily ration; we must have thousands of tons of it without delay." On another occasion Pershing was quoted as declaring, "You ask me what we need to win this war. I answer tobacco as much as bullets."[4]

Another source reported that in 1885 cigarettes comprised only one percent of the tobacco industry (which included chewing tobacco, cigars, pipes, snuff, and so forth). Five years later sales had risen 50 percent. However, even though cigarettes were only a tiny part of the tobacco industry an opposition had formed and was very active by then. There was no such lobbying against cigars, or pipes though, for example. And generally, laws that prohibited the sale of cigarettes did not prohibit the sales of other forms of tobacco. In 1892 cigarettes were labeled by the U.S. Senate Committee on Epidemic Diseases to be "an evil" and a "public hazard and urged petitioners to seek remedies from states," after being prodded by anti-cigarette forces. They claimed that federal officials had no jurisdiction in the matter, only the states did.[5]

John L. Sullivan, boxing folk hero of the late 19th century, served as a spokesman for his times when he dismissed the cigarette as a smoke suitable for "dudes and college misfits" and decidedly un–American, a reference to the foreign origin of both the tobacco leaf used in many brands and the immigrant masses favoring them, especially in New York. As late as 1910, wrote Richard Kluger, New York accounted for 25 percent of all the cigarettes sold in the United States. Men of substance and virility smoked cigars, he added. Besides paupers, only the effeminate, the effete, or the affected chose cigarettes, according to the charges leveled against them.[6]

Virginia Ernster wrote that at the start of the 20th century cigarette smoking was socially unacceptable for women but was gaining a foothold with men, who still showed a preference for cigars with the former having long been deemed a feminine object compared to the cigar. In the mid–19th century, said Ernster, it was considered poor taste for gentlemen to smoke in public during hours when women might be encountered, and at the end of the 1800s, women could not join their male counterparts in the smoking room after dinner, even in private gatherings. It was written of this period, "Between the lips of a woman [the cigarette] was generally regarded as no less than a badge of questionable character."[7]

In 1884 the *New York Times* declared: "The cigarette is designed for boys and women. The decadence of Spain began when the Spaniards adopted cigarettes, and if this pernicious practice obtains among adult Americans the ruin of the Republic is close at hand."[8]

It was against this backdrop in the 1880s that the issue of women smoking cigarettes moved to the forefront and began to grab the attention of the media, the general public, and reformers.

3

Abroad, 1880–1908

"A fumeuse may frequently make herself additionally inter-
esting and piquante."
— Anonymous French woman, 1888

"Smoking in some of the most reputable [English] restau-
rants is common, especially if a woman is accompanied by
her husband or brother."
— Elizabeth Biddle, 1906

Cigarette smoking began earlier in Europe than it did in the United States. As a result, those foreign women were often criticized for being a poor example and blamed for the spread of the habit to America. Although what little smoking had taken place prior to this period seemed more or less distributed through all classes of society, such was not the case in this period. Overwhelmingly the smoking women of this period, abroad and in the United States, were held to be of the upper class. As early as 1874, a newspaper account remarked that in Europe and America tobacco was almost universally used, and it was said that among "the most aristocratic young ladies of the principal cities of Europe, there are many of them who smoke their cigarettes secretly, as regularly as the men do their pipes and cigars."[1]

Five years later an account spoke of the link between smoking and morality. After a particular court case in London had ended, a reporter commented, regarding the evidence in that case, that he was at a loss to understand why the practice of cigarette smoking among ladies "seems to be generally regarded by counsel as the usual accompaniment of, or pre-lude to immorality." He argued he would not have been astonished if that was a conclusion held by the "ignorant and narrow-minded among us," but he was surprised to find over and over again "enlightened" men who must have sometimes "found themselves in the company of ladies irreproachable in character, and who yet may have occasionally taken a whiff at a cigarette — pandering to the prejudices of the millions." Then the reporter digressed to a similar court case he recalled from a few years earlier wherein the evidence showed that a female was in the habit of smoking in the stable in the company of a favorite groom. "A shudder ran through the whole court; and the smoking seemed to be more objected to, on the score of morality, than the groom." Despite that he remarked that continental European customs had crept into England and smoking by women was then looked on much more leniently than it had been 15 years earlier (around 1864). Cigarette-smoking women were not immoral, he concluded.[2]

By the late 1880s, the habit was entrenched enough that it had developed a set of rules to guide a new convert through the practice and still be mindful of etiquette. A woman smoker in Paris (styled as a "fumeuse") had drawn up a set of rules for the use of the weed. However, some of the rules struck a London reporter as "rather peculiar," and he wondered if it was necessary to insist on their observance. "Never, never smoke in a restaurant or out of doors, even when in company with your husband," was one of the rules, as was "Never light a cigarette after 5 o'clock tea, even if your most intimate friends only are present. Smoke after your meals at home, either in a room ad hoc or in your boudoir." Another piece of advice was to not hold a cigarette between one's teeth or at the sides of one's mouth, as such "low tricks" were even unworthy of well-bred men, "and you must be mindful to carry the cigarette gracefully to your lips, and to blow gentle wreaths of etherized essence around you from your mouth, or if you like, down from your nose." By attending to these rules, exclaimed the compiler, "a fumeuse may frequently make herself additionally interesting and piquante." Another potential benefit was "blowing clouds of smoke from the nose may even develop into a most fascinating operation, provided the smoker has a pretty proboscis, and that the profile of it only be seen by the admiring cavalier or suitor as the blue-gray vapor descends delicately from the nostrils."[3]

Novelists were said to be including smoking women in their works, a sure sign of a trend. One 1893 report felt that the prominence of cigarette-smoking females in modern fiction, especially in respect to continental European upper-class women, was likely greater than was the practice in real life. Yet he admitted, "There is no question that cigarette smoking is common among the 'fine ladies' of Europe and particularly in the class from which [novelist] Marion Crawford has drawn some of his recent characters."[4]

Later that same year, with respect to England, it was declared that the habit had "unquestionably gained ground in marked degree among women of the ultra fashionable set within the past few years." Commenting on the increased consumption of tobacco by women, the *Cigar and Tobacco World* publication of London asserted that smoking among fashionable English women was quite the "proper thing." So great had been the change of popular opinion toward users of the weed, argued a journalist, that the social canons of England no longer forbade the use of cigarettes as "disgusting or unsuitable for women."[5]

An American woman (unnamed) wrote to the European edition of the *New York Herald* on the subject of women smoking, also in 1893. The question of whether or not to smoke was an issue talked about in feminine circles. An English magazine had featured two articles on the topic, pro and con, in its October 1893 issue. Lady Colin Campbell was in favor of the habit, while Mrs. Lynn Linton opposed the practice, calling it "unwomanly." In any case, the American woman said it was becoming quite a common thing for women in England to smoke. Her attention was first drawn to the fact that women were beginning to smoke at a dinner party at a very "smart house." Present were half a dozen young women, all married. When the party was assembled in the drawing room, coffee and cigarettes were passed around. She was the only woman there who declined the latter "and was evidently considered a Goth. I must confess that as I glanced at each pretty mouth puffing out smoke as the owner lolled back in her chair, in a regular smoker's attitude, I did not think it added to her attractions in my eyes." When the husbands rejoined the group they looked on the scene as a matter of course; they seemed to be used to it. The American woman added that "respectable looking" girls could be seen coming out of London tobacco shops with lit cigarettes in their mouths. Also, at the Earl's Court exhibition, and even at the Imperial Institute grounds, "ladies enjoy the weed in public."[6]

As the 1890s progressed, the cigarette habit was said to have spread to women all over the world, during the previous few years. A French observer thought that one reason why that was happening in his country, where the cigarette habit was "extending among young women of the most exclusive circles," was due to the association of men and women in all kinds of sports. That had led to a greater degree of intimacy between the sexes, and "even the most critical no longer protest when two rosy lips send out a few puffs of smoke between a couple of games of tennis." Going higher up the class ladder revealed that even nobles and royalty engaged in the practice. The empress of Austria smoked 30–40 cigarettes a day; the dowager empress of Russia smoked (but only in her private apartments, apparently in deference to the sensibilities of the young czarina, who opposed the use of cigarettes) while the queen of Romania, the queen regent of Spain, Queen Amalia of Portugal (who followed her mother's example), the queen of Italy, and the wife of the Comte de Paris were all confirmed smokers. As well, Queen Victoria was reported to have a well-known fondness for snuff.[7]

Spread of the habit downward through the classes in England was noted in 1898 when the *Daily Telegraph* wrote about the "enormous" increase in the number of women smokers: "The great middle class is smoking as unconstrainedly as the aristocracy, and the working woman is fast following." Looking for an explanation for the increase, the newspaper declared that inquiries made among doctors, tobacconists, and others revealed, "the bicycle is responsible for much, as, with wheel parties, has arisen a freedom of manner unknown in the presence of chaperons."[8]

When a New Orleans businessman returned home in 1899 after a trip to London, he commented that he was greatly surprised at the number of women he saw smoking in public. While he thought one could always see such things in the bohemian resorts and the cafés patronized mainly by people from the continent, it was a shock for him to encounter such sights at posh establishments like the Savoy and Hotel Cecil. In both of those places, and three or four others equally aristocratic, he saw society women puffing away at cigarettes "as coolly as chappies at a roof garden." So common had such a spectacle become "that it has ceased to attract any attention, and it was tolerably evident that the ladies who were indulging did so because they liked it, and not merely to be eccentric."[9]

Another sign that the habit had caught on was the development of accessories to sell to those involved. One of the London tobacconists brought out a cigarette holder especially for women around 1900. It was made of a lemon-tinted amber, rimmed with gold. Not even the amber went into the mouth of the smoker, since a little quill was provided in the silver case that carried the holder, and that was placed in the mouth. Supposedly that method of use prevented any discoloration of the lips or fingers of the smoker.[10]

During a high-society dinner party in London in 1901 at the home of Lady De Gray, King Edward VII rebuked a noblewoman who was about to light a cigarette. To the king's rebuke, De Gray's guest answered, "Your Majesty, I'd rather die than not smoke." Replied the king: "Die, then, and smoke." Edward's rebuke was said to have created consternation among society women, "hundreds of whom are habitual smokers." Queen Alexandra (King Edward's wife) also was a smoker.[11]

In the opinion of the London *Telegraph* newspaper, for the previous

25 years society had looked on women and cigarettes with more toleration. One by one the fashionable restaurants had extended the same freedom of smoking after a meal to ladies as to gentlemen. The smoking room was then said to be a feature of all the ladies' clubs. Other signs of the spread and acceptance of the habit could be seen in the fact that gold cigarette cases could often be seen among the bride's presents at fashionable weddings, and not far from Bond Street there were tobacco shops that catered to female customers. But it was in the less aristocratic ranks that the real increase of women cigarette smokers was most marked, felt the newspaper. If one did not see much evidence of that in the streets, the report still argued, "There is no doubt that working women are beginning to smoke."[12]

Elizabeth Banks was described in 1902 as a special correspondent to the Sunday *Washington Post*. She sent back a report from London where one evening she went out to dinner with two unmarried female friends in their early 30s. Each was a professional woman who earned a good living. They went to a "cheap" Italian restaurant in the Soho area, a place frequented by actors, artists, journalists, and authors. After dinner and dessert, with the coffee, both the friends smoked cigarettes (Banks was a nonsmoker). She looked around the restaurant and saw a dozen other women smoking. Her reaction was that she felt "ashamed." Banks worried what would happen if some American man or woman, unfamiliar with English customs in the 20th century, should walk in and recognize her: "What would he think? What kind of associates would be think I had? ... Me in a restaurant sitting at a table with two other women — without the escort of a man — the two women smoking!" Later that evening she ran into an American male friend (just arrived from the United States that day) and told him of her "anger and shame" in the restaurant. He agreed with her and said if he had wandered into the restaurant and saw what Banks had described he would have been tempted to snub the smoker. "Drop those women. They can't be nice," he advised. Believing such a situation could only happen in those cheap Italian restaurants, the couple went on to one of the "smartest" restaurants in London, attached to one of the best hotels. However, he didn't take Banks in because he first looked in by himself and was horrified to see at least 20 women smoking cigarettes, all from high society and the nobility. Then they went to an in-between type restaurant. They did go in, but even there women were smoking. Banks's male friend also smoked there. Of the couple's experiences, Banks concluded: "He says he knew English women smoked, but he did not know they smoked in public restaurants. He is learning to be charitable and liberal. So am I, but I hate it — this smoking of women in restaurants."[13]

Author Mrs. Hugh Fraser (sister of novelist Marion Crawford and niece of Julia Ward Howe) was also something of a world traveler. In 1905 she sailed for Japan, but before she left she gave a public talk in Washington, D.C., about her travels abroad and told of the "universality" of the custom of smoking among upper-class women of all nationalities, except among Japanese women. Fraser admitted she had never seen one of that country's women of nobility smoke, nor had one ever told her that she indulged. Nonetheless, Fraser assumed they did so in their own homes but did not want to talk about it. Although she had seen no upper-class Japanese women smoke, she related that the middle- and lower-class females did so "constantly." With respect to other lands, Fraser declared that "all the upper class women abroad smoke — English, French, German, Italian and Russian. In many circles in England it is expected that cigarettes shall be passed to the women after dinner.... At after theater suppers one always smokes." All Russian women were said to smoke a great deal, and an upper-class Italian female would be surprised not to be offered a cigarette after dinner. Heaviest smokers of all, she thought, were the Austrian women — who smoked cigars.[14]

On the window of one of the first-class carriages of a train that left London for Liverpool on the morning of March 21, 1906, was displayed a label that read "Ladies' Smoking." The carriage that held that sign was the first women's smoking car ever run on an English railway and thought to be the first in the world. It was occupied by a small party of women for whom it had been reserved. An application for such a carriage was made by a man on March 20; the railway decided to comply. Three women were in the reservation party, and "they started smoking as soon as they were seated."[15]

Journalist Elizabeth Biddle did not think the railroad car for women smokers was such a big deal. English women frequently smoked on their rail journeys, she explained, if a party of friends were in a compartment by themselves. Of course, it was against the rules to smoke except in the smoking compartments, but English railroad rules were often stretched or ignored completely. A woman or man who wanted to smoke in a non-smoking carriage could do so, provided the other occupants did not object or complain.[16]

Biddle observed that by then (1906), in England it had long ceased to be a matter for comment when a woman smoked either privately or publicly. By privately she did not mean on the sly, for she had never known of an English woman who made a secret of the fact that she was a smoker. In her view, that was the chief way in which she differed from the American woman smoker for in the United States it was still considered not "the thing" for a woman to take a cigarette, so the American woman hid her use of tobacco, or tried to. English women smoked because they liked it, explained Biddle. They did not look on the practice as smart or fast, neither immoral nor objectionable. "If you are under the impression that it is 'devilish' to smoke your ideas are so provincial," Biddle told her readers. "Those who do smoke do not conceal it or labor under the impression that they are either chic or degenerate." Around 12 years earlier, Biddle had seen women smoking for the first time at a reception of arts people in London. She was offered a cigarette herself but was embarrassed. Some half dozen women were smoking in the room, which caused Biddle to worry she "had got into a crowd which was not exactly 'nice.'" Many of her English married women friends told her they would never have thought of smoking until their husband suggested it for the sake of companionship and good comradeship. For Biddle, one English anomaly was that an unmarried girl or woman in good society did not usually go out with a man unchaperoned. She could, though, smoke a cigarette with him. Biddle concluded, "Smoking in some of the most reputable restaurants is common, especially if a woman is accompanied by her husband or brother."[17]

Another London newspaper, the *Chronicle*, published a piece in 1906 about the large increase in women smokers then under way. Ten or fifteen years earlier, it felt, smoking among females had been more or less confined to isolated cases of young girls who thought it clever or amusing and elderly females of the tramp class. By 1906, though, it was much different, with women smokers being found in every class of the community: students, society women, shop girls, journalists, artists, businesswomen, young girls, married women, and even grandmothers. At the same time as women smokers were increasing, men were said to be becoming more tolerant and more used to the sight of women with cigarettes.[18]

Yet that *Chronicle* article went on to list in great detail the reasons why women should not smoke. The main argument put forward was that women were more extreme than men. What might be moderate smoking for a man could be dangerously near excess for a young girl. "A man may smoke a dozen cigarettes in twenty-four hours without any apparent damage to his health, the girl who habitually disposes of six or eight cigarettes a day is deliberately undermining her constitution," went the argument. One of the first duties of a woman, explained the account, was to preserve her health; "because, in spite of all the assertions and indignant denials by the shrieking sisterhood, the chief reason for our very existence is to provide the mothers of future generations." Added the author, "and there is no more pathetic figure than the heavy smoker of the gentler sex. Thin, anemic, highly strung, irritable, with cold, clammy hands, and stained fingertips, she is one of the least admirable products of the woman movement." According to this account, nervous symptoms resulting from smoking would be more apparent in a woman smoker than in a man because a woman's nervous organization was of a more delicate order and was more easily upset. As a final thought, the reporter believed that to smoke in a public place laid a woman open to the criticism of strangers, and while a female was not necessarily "fast" because she had an occasional cigarette, "the true gentlewoman avoids doing anything unconventional in public. If a girl will smoke she should only do so among friends, in the privacy of her own house and, preferably, in a gathering of women who smoke themselves."[19]

While it was becoming more common for women in London to be seen smoking in public establishments in the first few years of the 20th century, the odd holdout could still be found. One of London's most exclusive women's clubs, the Ladies Park Club, moved into new premises in the summer of 1907. On that occasion it was noted that the club was believed to be the only West End club that strictly forbade bridge playing and smoking anywhere on its premises. Supposedly those prohibitions were used by the club as a means of excluding the "bad form smart set" and attracting "genuine gentlewomen."[20]

Special inquiries and surveys made by the London *Daily Telegraph* in 1908 purported to show that "four out of five of all English women of [social] position are smokers." (That was certainly highly exaggerated.) The account also claimed that "every restriction" against the woman smoker had finally been removed at all the fashionable London hotels and restaurants. Said the manager of a West End hotel, "Of course any woman dining alone who started to smoke would be asked to desist, but no woman dines alone. Women dine only with men or in companies. When cigars are passed to the men, cigarettes are passed to the women." Cigarette smoking among women was said to not be limited to any particular class and that nobody with even a modicum of sophistication "pays the slightest attention to the question whether women are smoking in public or not. Nobody cares." Another observer declared that women of all ages smoked after lunch, tea, and dinner, and still another observer said that factory girls were the only females who then regarded the cigarette as "vulgar." Most inveterate smokers were said to be the suffragettes, as those women tried to outsmoke men. Looking further afield to other nations, this piece stated that Russian, German, Danish, Austrian, Polish, Egyptian, Spanish, and Japanese women smoked. However, Italian women hardly ever smoked, and French women, except for artists, writers, politicians, and students, smoked very little. American women were said to smoke the least of all.[21]

4
America, 1880–1908

*"It doesn't seem to be very womanly ... I wouldn't for the
world have my boy see me with a cigarette in my mouth."*
— Mrs. Thurber, 1894

*"American ideas will not be shocked by the conjunction of
a cigarette and a woman in public."*
— Anonymous New York City
restaurant owner, 1897

*"The general sentiment among our women is that for women
to smoke is vulgar."*
— Harper's Weekly, 1900

Writing in the *Washington Post* in 1888, a reporter declared that any
talk about women smoking in the nation's capital was very much exaggerated. However, it was admitted there were numbers of Cubans, Spaniards and some French women "of beauty and position" in Washington who
bought cigarettes in person, smoked them at dinners, and offered them to
female friends in their bedrooms. "But they are only importing a foreign
custom, which does not strike any strong root here," asserted the account.[1]

Later in that same year, an account about the situation in New York
City painted a quite different picture. Noted was that the habit of cigarette smoking was growing very common there among the women with
users coming from all grades of society; many did it "constantly," while
many more took an occasional cigarette "by way of good-fellowship with
other women" who were smoking. Yet there were lines that the female
puffer did not cross at that time, for the piece stated, "I don't mean to
assert that it is seen in public at all. No woman smokes on the street, nor
in conveyances, either public or private." Where they did smoke was in
"very many of the best houses." When the women at social affairs at these

21

houses left the men to their wine after dinner and went to the drawing room, the footman brought in the coffee for the women. On his tray he had a box of Egyptian or Turkish cigarettes and a box of matches. "Not all the women take them, but those who do not are not shocked at those who do. It is no longer considered fast," explained the reporter. In novelty shops at the time, among other Christmas goods, were reported to be smoking sets for women — items containing cigarette holders and cases with compartments for cigarettes, matches, and so on.[2]

According to a report from an 1890 issue of the Philadelphia *Times*, women who played poker seldom smoked while the most "ardent devotees" of the cigarette were found among "busy" women.[3]

From Boston came an 1891 report in which it was declared that cigarette smoking among women was said to be "alarmingly" on the increase. Those who had acquired the habit were described as usually being women who moved in very good society with it being "much more common among the upper than the middle classes." However, in a contradictory fashion the piece added: "women leading low lives are almost always confirmed smokers of this noxious form of the weed." In the description of a single example it was observed that people passing a fashionable apartment house in Boston's Beacon Hill area used to see around dusk every day a young woman seated in a window puffing a cigarette "with the air of an easy abandon." She blew the smoke through her nose "with the dreamy air of one rendered oblivious to surroundings through intense enjoyment." Though it used to be a rare thing for women to openly purchase cigarettes at tobacco shops in Boston, by 1901 such transactions were said to be too frequent to cause much comment.[4]

A reporter writing under the name of Mrs. M'Guirk surveyed Washington, D.C.'s leading society women in 1894 to see what their attitude was to the habit and to find out how many of them were smokers. Mrs. Romero (wife of the Mexican ambassador) said she did not smoke herself; that she had never seen ladies smoking in Washington, though she admitted to having heard that some did indulge; and that she would never offer cigarettes to women in her own home because she did not think it was "womanly." Romero concluded, of the practice: "I don't believe you will find it very prevalent in Washington, for I can truthfully say that I have never been offered a cigarette in all the time I have lived here." Emphatic in declaring she did not approve of smoking was Mrs. Lamont, who added she would never encourage the practice of offering anyone cigarettes and that she never would use them herself. Lamont admitted that at the houses of some of her closest friends the women did use cigarettes. "When we were in Washington before I saw ladies smoking, but only in rare instances and then the woman had acquired the habit abroad," she added. "You know that is where our girls learn to tolerate it." M'Guirk mentioned Mrs. de Struve (wife of the Russian ambassador in Washington, although the couple seemed to be no longer stationed in Washington at the time of the account). Mrs. de Struve was described as a person who always smoked after dinner, no matter where she was. Whether she was in her own house or someone else's, she always went back to the dining room for a cigarette. During the time she was in Washington, everyone in capital society was said to have referred to her habit "and the tone in which some of them describe the sang froid with which she calmly lit her cigarette in the houses of some very straight-laced people is strongly tinctured with admiration for her audacity."[5]

M'Guirk also spoke to Mrs. Oley, who acknowledged she had heard of ladies smoking but was adamant in stating they would not get any cigarettes in her home. She had seen females smoking abroad and felt that after that, somehow, the habit did not seem to be quite such an offense. "Most of the American women who do use cigarettes, I think, contract the habit abroad, but I'm sure it hasn't made any great progress, no matter what is said, among women in this country," concluded Lamont. Miss Herbert assured M'Guirk she would never smoke herself nor would she ever provide cigarettes for ladies in her own home. Positive that all "womanly women" were opposed to their sex taking any active interest in cigarettes was Mrs. Hoke Smith. She did not think men liked to see their wives with cigarettes between their lips or with stained fingers, and that would be sufficient in itself to keep the cigarette "peculiarly the adjunct of men." One woman who expressed a personal antipathy to tobacco was Mrs. Thurber (wife of President Grover Cleveland's private secretary), who disapproved of smoking by anybody, not just by women. "I disapprove of it from every standpoint. It doesn't seem to be womanly ... I don't think it is attractive in any way whatever," she exclaimed. Thurber also knew women who smoked. "Then, too, I should have to oppose it as the mother of children whom I hope will not be smokers; yes, as a mother I should be most strongly opposed to my children seeing women smoke," she offered as another objection and added, "I wouldn't for the world have my boy see me with a cigarette in my mouth." All of those opinions caused M'Guirk to conclude that although those "representative" women ranged themselves against females smoking, they all had friends, presumably their equals, who not only believed differently, but put those beliefs into practice.[6]

Another report from 1894, about New York City, argued there were probably fewer American society women who were smokers (and drinkers) than media accounts might have led one to believe. That is, an exaggerated emphasis was placed on the subject by media outlets. A female physician with an extensive practice in that city was asked if she knew habitual smokers and drinkers among American women of "the higher classes." She replied "No. I have never had cultivated women appeal to me for help from such habits, nor do I know one woman so afflicted." Then a "prominent" society woman of New York was asked the same question. Admitting she knew several women who smoked and drank habitually, she explained, "but they are not the kind that one cares to know intimately. They show their small vices as a revolt against Puritanism, which they detest." Next, a woman who had been on the stage for several years was queried. Arguing she had never met an American woman who drank heavily, she allowed that cigarettes were favored by a few that she knew. These interviews caused the reporter to declare that smokers were rare, even among the most fashionable women, or else "such failings would be more conspicuous." Speculating about the origins of the habit, no matter how rare it may have been, he declared: "Unquestionably, the influences at work are foreign, and, even if they affect but a small portion of our society, should we not question soberly the wisdom of their suppression?" Being just a seven-day journey from Europe he felt it was inevitable "that its unprofitable customs and vices should be brought to us continually, but we need not bring them in ourselves."[7]

Blame for the fad was assigned differently a year later by a reporter in the nation's capital. In that account it was the fault of the "new woman." She rode a bicycle, had no objection to the "ever offending" bloomers, understood the income tax, knew all about the tariff, believed in dress reform, discoursed on the suffrage issue, "but her very latest and likewise her most appalling fad is smoking." Reportedly this new woman was no longer content to smoke in the privacy of her own bedroom, indulging in a quiet after-dinner smoke, but smoked openly and above board, asserting she had as much right to the use of the weed as her brother or husband. Two of the young matrons in the Dupont Circle area of Washington were described as enjoying twilight smokes each evening on their front door steps, "and between the puffs hold the cigarettes in their white jeweled fingers in the most approved manner." Some sort of "smoking guild" was in existence with the new women members meeting occasionally at the home of a popular matron, who also enjoyed "hitting the cigarette."[8]

New York City almost certainly had more smokers per capita in the 1890s than any other U.S. city. According to an 1895 piece, which acknowledged New York's lead, Chicago had not then taken up the habit. Said the account: "To be sure, a few society lights are believed to indulge in this species of dissipation in the sacred privacy of the boudoir, but the prac-

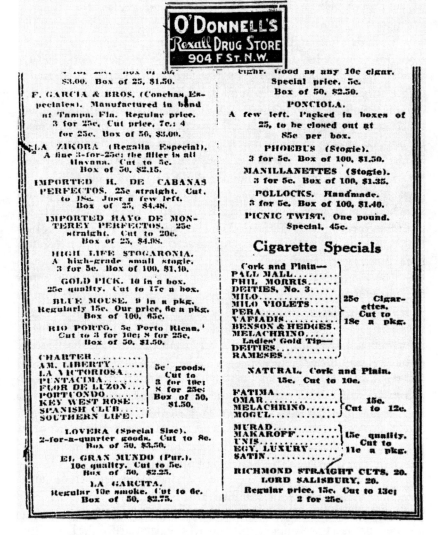

A 1915 ad for tobacco from a Washington, D.C., drug store. Note in the right-hand column, two-thirds of the way down, a mention for a brand specifically for women. Cigarette brands for women were a not uncommon feature of the early 1900s, but none were successful.

tice has been condemned by others whose words carry great weight. Consequently the habit is slow to take root and may never become common" in Chicago. Arguing that smoking among New York women had long been common in secret before London gave the practice its stamp of approval, the reporter offered as one reason for a increased female consumption the

availability of "dainty" cigarettes—brands made especially for women—
"miniature editions of what man carries." The cigarettes in the women's
brands were thinner and shorter than the standard smokes bought by men.
Containing much less tobacco, they cost relatively much more than the
brands that men bought. Such women's cigarettes, made from good-quality
Turkish tobacco retailed at around $3 to $3.50 per hundred cigarettes,
although some went as high as $5 or $6. Cheaper brands, with lower-grade
tobacco, were available, running as low as $1 per hundred. Specially made
brands of cigarettes for women were minor parts of the scene up to around
World War I. However, they never really caught on. A woman newly con-
verted to smoking might have started with such a brand—attracted by the
package, and so on, which was designed to appeal to women—but quickly
switched to buying the standard brands that men favored and bought. The
most likely reason was that the women's brands were relatively a poor buy.
One critic referred to them derogatorily as "three puffs and out," a reference to their very puny size.[9]

Contradicting the above reference to Chicago was an account a year
later, in 1896. A manicurist in that city was cited as saying more women
were smoking there as she had a steady stream of customers with tobacco-
stained fingers. "Women smoke assiduously at home, until their fingers
are as yellow as parchment, and then they come here to have the evidence
of their vice removed," she explained. A large percentage of her patrons
had regular weekly appointments to have the inside points of the thumb
and index fingers cleaned of nicotine. Those smokers were reported to
have given up the "dainty, perfumed Turkish cigarettes" for the stronger
and cheaper American product, which decreased their cost from five cents
per cigarette down to one cent each. That increase in consumption was
found in society women in Chicago, not other classes.[10]

Journalist Helen Bullitt Lowry, writing in 1921 about the late 1890s,
noted that smoking for women, unlike the shimmy dance, "has come down
in the world to the bourgeoisie instead of up in the world from the demi-
monde." It was a by-product of high society, which learned the habit from
Europe. Around 1896, she wrote, the first female cigarette smoker appeared
on the horizon of America—if one did not count the pipe smokers found
in the mountains of Tennessee. Lowry referred to Baroness de Struve.
When she produced a cigarette at her first diplomatic dinner, the other
guests did not call it "fast" then; they described it as "mannish." De Struve
stayed in the dining room with the men and joined the women after smoking. According to Lowry, cigarettes were well established in diplomatic
circles among the wives of American ambassadors returned from foreign
parts, long before American society at home took up the habit. In her view,

the chorus girl, the matinee-going middle-class woman and the flappers had learned the habit from the upper class U.S. society women, and the practice was spreading every day.[11]

Harper's Weekly observed in 1900, "reputable and well-mannered American women rarely smoke nowadays ... The general sentiment among our women is that for women to smoke is vulgar." Uncertain as to why that was so, the magazine declared: "All we know is that as a rule men smoke and women don't."[12]

Still, the practice increased in America. When Chicago-based *Zeal*, the organ of the Federation of Young People's Societies, surveyed the situation, it described cigarette smoking among women as having grown to be a "menace" in the United States. The publication cited a cigarette manufacturer as saying that in New York City his firm had 10,000 "ladies of the highest class of society" as regular patrons (it was not uncommon then for people to buy cigarettes by mail from a tobacco shop or even a manufacturer). Several of his regular retail customers bought from 500 to 1,000 cigarettes each month to sell to women. In San Francisco ten women smoked to every one in Chicago, reportedly, and it was the same in New York City (ten to one over Chicago). A second cigarette manufacturer was cited as having claimed there were 100,000 women in New York City who smoked. And "In Pittsburgh, Philadelphia, Albany, Buffalo — in fact in all the Eastern cities, with the exception of Washington — it is the rule rather than the exception for society women to indulge in the use of tobacco in this form."[13]

More anecdotal evidence about the increase of the habit in Chicago came from one of that city's leading dentists, who commented in 1904 that he had more and more patients with discolored teeth. One of those patients told him that smoking was not uncommon among women who played bridge, while many of the younger set dallied with the weed but had not yet become "cigarette fiends." Among tobacconists in Chicago, it was admitted that the sale of cigarettes to women of all classes had been increasing. Most women were said to buy the imported (more expensive) cigarettes, but the confirmed, "utterly gone" smokers used a cheaper grade made from Virginia tobacco (standard America-made brands purchased by men) that contained "plenty of ocherish stain and is all the worse for the teeth and nerves." Many of Chicago's smart set then smoked, and some of those sported cigarette cases elaborately designed and often studded with jewels. With respect to the attitude of males to females smoking, it was reported that some took broad and tolerant views, whereas others were unable to reconcile the cigarette habit "with their ideals of womanly grace and perfection."[14]

Whatever the prevalence of cigarette-smoking women may have been in the first few years of the 20th century, enough interest and attention was generated that advice articles started to appear. One came from Julian Hawthorne in 1903. If you thought it was wrong for yourself, then it was wrong, he stated, but if one did it only out of bravado, then that woman was a "vulgar hussy." However, "if you possess the greatness to be truly indifferent to outside opinion, or if you are so sincerely innocent as not to suspect yourself of audacity, you may safely produce your cigarette in the drawing room of Lady Pharisee herself." Hawthorne remarked that in many foreign lands many women smoked with confidence because they were backed by public opinion and the custom of their country. "But now and then one of these chastened libertines strays from her native land, and finds her way to us, bringing her country's custom with her, and she, in her naïve pursuance of her habit, acts the part, no doubt of an efficient missionary of the weed."[15]

Marie Studholme was another with an advice article in 1904. In answer to her own question as to whether women should smoke, she said a woman should if she really liked it. However, Studholme argued that very few women honestly did enjoy the habit; not more than one in ten was her estimate. "They pretend to; but, as a rule, a woman only smokes because she considers it a smart, up-to-date thing to do. It is not, all the same." She predicted it was a fad among women that, like cycling, would fade away and that we would never see a woman — at least an American woman — smoking in public. "I have once or twice seen one with a cigarette in a hansom cam; but it is rare, and I hope it will continue to be so. It would look horrible — absolutely horrible — to see women on buses and trains smoking," she added. "It would be neither pretty nor piquant, merely vulgar and most masculine; and I am sure no man would approve of a woman smoking if she carried it to such a length as that." Despite all she had said, Studholme ended her article by confessing: "Of course, I smoke myself — just a little. Sometimes when I'm worried, or want to think something over quietly, then I bring out my cigarette case and have a puff or two."[16]

As a companion piece to Studholme's was one on the same page by Dr. Alexander Barton, a physician. In answer to the same question Studholme had asked herself Barton replied, "I think not. Personally, I never care to see a woman with a cigarette in her mouth. It is neither graceful nor womanly." Although the format of the two articles was the pro/con style, and they answered the same question yes/no, Studholme's piece could hardly be viewed as in favor of smoking. After the initial yes, the article was entirely negative about the topic. Barton went on to declare that the average man did not care to see women smoking, certainly not in public.

"It is far too masculine-looking to please his taste — a fact overlooked by many women," he explained. "They seem to forget that smoking is extremely masculine, and that once a girl earns for herself the title of 'masculine' she has lost much of her charm from a man's point of view. Men detest masculine women, only women don't seem to realize the fact."[17]

A survey about women's tobacco usage in Washington, D.C., was conducted by a reporter in 1906. One tobacco dealer told him he had no doubt the habit was increasing "enormously," but that proof of the increase was hard to come by. One reason was because the "better class" of women who smoked never went into tobacco shops to buy their own cigarettes. Rather, they sent in a male relative or a servant to purchase smokes for them. Continuing his survey, the reporter declared that investigations at one after another of the leading tobacco stores in Washington revealed the same sentiments. They all said that some of the women came into the shop nonchalantly and purchased their particular brand "as if they were getting newspapers," while some were very cautious, "coming in with numerous backward glances to insure against detection." Still, the reporter admitted he could provide no real proof of the phenomenon because "there are no cafés which permit smoking among the ladies, and there are no clubs which have a ladies' smoking room. As yet there are no smoking cars on the trains that run into Washington, but the dealers here all shake their heads knowingly and declare that the women are getting more and more under the influence of tobacco." Within the previous year it was said the big department stores in Washington had almost doubled their regular supply of ladies' cigarette cases. Also, the smaller tobacco shops all carried a regular line of women's brands of smokes although it was acknowledged they were not often called for, "as the women prefer the same brands that the men use."[18]

A year later, in 1907, an article on the increasing number of women smokers was published and also dealt with the question of finding evidence for the trend. That there were more users was vouched for by tobacco dealers, beauticians, hairdressers, and certain physicians. Some light was also shed on the issue after a scare that was caused by the announcement that after a certain date cigarettes could not be sold legally in Illinois. Shortly after that false rumor was printed in newspapers, tobacco dealers were "flooded" with phone calls from women to see if the rumor was true. Dealers became more convinced that some of the cigarettes purchased at their outlets by men were not all consumed by men. As in Washington, the Chicago dealers believed very few female users purchased their own cigarettes. Beauticians were aware of cigarette usage because of the odor on customers' breaths when they visited beauty shops. Some of those establishments had operators whose duty was to remove cigarette stains from the fingers of patrons. Cited as another proof of the existence and extent of female smoking was said to be the presence on department store counters of complete cigarette smoking outfits designed especially for and used largely by women.[19]

Chicago physicians on house calls often found evidence of smoking women who reportedly became "indignant" when the medical men ordered them to give up cigarettes. "Always they deny that they have used tobacco in any form," went the account, "but the doctors say that excessive cigarette smoking never fails to leave its peculiar effect on the heart action, and that they seldom are deceived by those who try to make them believe that they never smoke." Dr. Frank Heron believed cigarette smoking had spread to a remarkable extent among women "and especially among the better class of women." Druggists and beauticians had made it possible for a woman to smoke cigarettes without being detected by anyone besides her physician, said Heron, because the beauticians removed the stains from the fingers and the druggists sold them preparations to sweeten their breath. Several tobacco shops on Chicago's west side were said to cater especially to women's smoking needs. None of the downtown tobacco shops, however, could estimate the extent of the habit because the cigarettes consumed by them were seldom bought directly by them. Yet all those dealers agreed that the habit was on the increase and that most of the female smokers were from "the fashionable world."[20]

Public Places

Although most smoking by women in this period took place in private with the user consuming in the privacy of her own home or at gatherings, dinners, parties, and so on, of a private nature, mainly among the upper classes, the movement to take the habit to public places was under way. Europe, of course, moved farther and faster in that direction than did America. In 1897 men were allowed to smoke after dinner in Delmonico's restaurant, following the leads of other high-class New York City restaurants that adopted the European custom and permitted smoking (apparently the first establishment to allow men to smoke did so in 1883). But, said the report, as of 1897 women had never been allowed to smoke in any of the New York first-class restaurants, "in spite of the fact that scarcely a day passed without an effort in that direction." The "indignant" women who were usually interrupted just as they were about to light a smoke were "almost invariably foreigners, and their protests against the discrimination are invariably eloquent and spirited. But in no case has an exception been made." A proprietor of one restaurant explained to a reporter, "American ideas will not be shocked by the conjunction of a cigarette and a woman in public." New York restaurants were not, like some of the best-known ones in London, supplied with smoking rooms especially for women.[21]

In the dining room of one of the posh hotels uptown in New York City in 1904, an engraved card was placed on the tables at the dinner hour that read: "Gentlemen and ladies wishing to smoke may do so in the gilt-room." That room was back of the parlor on the second floor and every evening there, according to an account, "may be seen a score of handsomely dressed women smoking Turkish cigarettes in company with the men."[22]

An editorial in the *New York Times* in December 1907 commented that it was not news that cigarette smoking by women was not tolerated in the public rooms of the city's hotels and restaurants. Said the editor: "Women who smoke cigarettes in public are still generally accounted vulgar, if not actually wicked." He added, "No thoroughly sophisticated American woman of good breeding would think of lighting a cigarette in a New York restaurant." In conclusion he declared, "The managers of our hotels are to be commended for prohibiting cigarette smoking by women, because they are acting in accord with public opinion."[23]

All of that was about to change, at least in one instance. One feature of the New Year's celebration on December 31, 1907, in the Times Square area of New York was that smoking by women was permitted in Martin's, one of the most celebrated restaurants. It had been announced publicly that this new policy could be expected and women did smoke there that night and "nobody looked shocked, and few if any were." Permission to smoke was presented as this restaurant's New Year's gift to its female patrons. It was noted that male smokers were barred from very few New York restaurants at that time. "There is not a room at the Plaza or Sherry's in which [male] diners may not smoke." Also noted was that at least one other smart restaurant had allowed women to smoke once in a while, as the staff turned a blind eye to the practice.[24]

A few days later in a long interview, John B. Martin, proprietor of Café Martin, said, "It is not true that we are prepared to permit women to smoke openly." He said he would be happy to do so if at least a few other restaurants joined in, but he did not want to do it alone. Martin added that in Europe, where he spent his summers, "One thinks no more of seeing a woman smoke than of seeing her drink a glass of wine. Here women are permitted to drink a cocktail without comment, and yet the cocktail certainly has more power for harm than a cigarette. The truth is, it is all in the way it is done." Elaborating, Martin explained that if a "respected" woman came to his place with her husband and cared to join him in a cigarette, "we would not request her to stop, but if a conspicuous young woman started blowing rings of smoke simply for show we would promptly tell her it was not allowed, and ask her to go to the smoking room reserved for women on the second floor." Trying to clarify the situation Martin told the reporter his restaurant would countenance it in some cases, but with decided restrictions, as a whole. He did not want to make the thing common and was not sure the time was ripe for such a policy, but he was certain that if his place did start the custom others would follow.[25]

Recalling his start in the restaurant business, Martin reminisced that when he started the old Café Martin in 1883 (located in Lafayette Place), his success was rooted principally in the fact he allowed men to smoke in the dining rooms. At that time, 25 years earlier, the leading hotels and restaurants were in that neighborhood; including Delmonico's, the Hoffman House, the Hotel Brunswick, the St. James, and the Fifth Avenue Hotel. If men were dining with friends and cared to smoke, they had to excuse themselves and go into another room. That proved to be awkward for the women (females did not sit alone in restaurants) and as a consequence, said Martin, many people came to his place. Smoking by men was then general (1907) and accepted everywhere, added Martin. "Doubtless I will also start the custom of [women] smoking in New York, but I don't like to take up a question of so much importance single-handed," mused the restaurateur. "And yet some day when I feel like it I may say, 'All right; women may smoke. It is settled forever.' I'll be glad when I have the nerve to say that." During his travels he had seen women in Paris smoking in the Ritz and the Elysee Palace; in London English women smoked in upscale places such as the Princess, Carlton, Savoy, and New Ritz restaurants. "These places are Meccas for Americans, who copy the foreign styles and customs as carefully as possible."[26]

Martin's contention that other restaurants in New York did indeed leave him alone in a policy of letting women smoke was backed up by a brief survey of some other fashionable eateries there. At Rector's, it was emphatically denied that cigarette smoking was openly allowed. Manager A. Miller explained, "It is a little early to start the custom but when we are convinced that the majority of our customers want it we will let the women smoke." Asked if he would permit a female to smoke then in Rector's, Miller responded, "Decidedly not, if we saw her." Mr. Muschenhein, an executive with the Hotel Astor said that so far they had little demand for smoking by women to be allowed. "So far there has been no occasion to take the subject up seriously. If others did we would probably join them." Waldorf-Astoria hotel assistant manager Mr. Marshall commented, "We have never given the question much thought because it is so seldom brought up." According to him, perhaps once in a six-month period an English woman unfamiliar with U.S. conditions would light up in one of the hotel's restaurants. "We tell her it is against the rules, and the matter ends in her frank apology," he explained. "We have never seen an American woman smoke here and so never have been obliged to ask an American to stop, although every one knows they smoke in their own homes."[27]

An even more difficult situation for the smoking woman was to puff publicly in the street. Florence Bergen, described as a "dashing young woman who follows the races," was arraigned in Police Court in Washington, D.C., on December 28, 1895, charged with "having disturbed the peace, quiet, and good order of the city by smoking a cigarette on Pennsylvania Avenue." At the arraignment Bergen was described as "jauntily attired," and while she sat in the dock "she shook her head saucily and winked at the prosecuting attorney." Judge Kimball sent her to the workhouse for 15 days.[28]

Bergen's case prompted a *Washington Post* editor to express "astonishment and regret" at the 15-day sentence. That a young woman "of any character" should be imprisoned for smoking a cigarette on the street troubled and distressed the newspaperman. He wondered why should "this foolish, wayward, and reckless young woman be treated as a criminal and subjected to the disgrace and obloquy of imprisonment." Trying to understand the situation, the editor remarked it was a matter of common knowledge that women smoke cigarettes; "the spectacle is a matter of every-day experience. In scores of fashionable houses in this city, beautiful and charming ladies, leaders in the fashionable route, indulge the practice constantly — and why not?" Was it then, he wondered, denied to the poor, the unknown, the friendless and the doubtful (Bergen was clearly from the lower class) "to do what their more fortunate sisters may do without reproach? Or have our police elevated themselves to the position of censores morum, and undertaken to say that what is permitted to the rich and fashionable indoors shall not be permitted to the obscure and the scant of means upon the public thoroughfares?"[29]

On a September night in 1904, two men and two women were riding in a car on New York's Fifth Avenue. One of the women was smoking a cigarette. At Thirtieth Street, bicycle policeman Rensselaer stopped the car and ordered the woman to stop smoking. "You can't do that on Fifth Avenue while I'm patrolling here," he reportedly said. Ignoring his demand, the woman took a drag, exhaled in the policeman's face and while doing so flicked cigarette ash in his direction. Then the car continued, with Rensselaer following. Protesting against being followed, the men said they were not doing anything wrong. More words were exchanged, then, at Thirty-Fifth Street the officer arrested one of them as being drunk and disorderly. At the station when the man was being booked the woman stated that she had smoked a cigarette "and I don't see that I was doing any harm. I have done it in many other places, and I don't see why they should object to it in New York. I think the policeman overstepped his authority ... I can't see why he didn't arrest me, for I seemed to be the whole cause of the trouble." She gave her particulars as, Mrs. William P. Orr of the Waldorf, actress.[30]

Medical Opinion

When medical opinions were advanced in this period on the effects of tobacco on women they tended, for the most part, to be positive. In the 1874 account on snuff, the reporter thought snuff dipping was very beneficial to the teeth and that the habit was often acquired from using snuff as a dentifrice. His extensive travels through the South and the Southwest convinced him that wherever the practice prevailed the teeth of the women "were beautifully white and singularly free from decay." Tobacco was also said here to have high antiseptic and detergent properties "and must exercise a beneficial influence in purifying the mouth."[31]

In an 1879 British account, a journalist related that he had been told by several "eminent" medical men that as a rule, tobacco was less injurious to the female constitution than to that of the male. Insomnia was referred to as a condition to which women were "peculiarly subject," with tobacco acting as a decided soother of irritable nerves. Then he told of the experience of a woman he knew who had suffered terribly from insomnia for years and had tried every narcotic remedy without effect. At last she was induced to try smoking and "the beneficial result was almost instantaneous."[32]

A magazine called the *Hospital* got into trouble in 1892 for advising women whose nerves "cannot bear the strain of small worries" to try smoking, if their doctors recommended it. Apparently many people were irritated by the advice. But a supporter of the plan, James Payn, argued it could not be denied by anyone "short of a fanatic" that a pipe allayed the troubles of a man; therefore why shouldn't a few puffs on a cigarette do the same for females? "At present its mitigations among the fair sex are confined chiefly to the fast and loose, but there is no reason why it should be so."[33]

An 1893 piece about England featured the comment that dentists had been aware for years that habitual users of cigarettes had the best preserved teeth, "tobacco being such an active germicide." Another health benefit was found in a report from Dr. Theodore Griffin, who claimed that in all his years of medical experience he had never seen a single case of consumption in a tobacco addict: "On the contrary, the rule has been that habitual smokers have good lungs." Because of those observations, Griffin advocated the practice of smoking by women become more general.[34]

An English doctor in 1904 was reported to thoroughly approve the use of tobacco "as not only harmless, but wholesome in counteracting some of the tendencies of high-pressure modern life." It was an attitude and belief that was blamed in this account for being at least partly responsible for the rapid spread of the cigarette habit among English women around that time.[35]

Dr. Martin, the city of Cleveland Health Officer, advised the women of Cleveland's "smart set" to smoke cigarettes in 1906. He had found that society women were addicted to the excessive use of tea, and he attributed to its abuse the spread of heart disease among them. Tea acted as a stimulant while nicotine depressed the heart, so that one counteracted the effect of the other, explained Martin.[36]

Not all medical reports from the period were positive, however, one was particularly ahead of its time. Commenting on a 1907 case, in one of the Baltimore hospitals of a female patient with a "tobacco heart" (a term regularly used then but only vaguely explained; it described, apparently, an increased heart rate, plus other symptoms) despite the fact she had never used the weed herself in any form. Baltimore Health Commissioner Dr. Bosley said that such a thing as a tobacco heart was, under the circumstances, not only possible but also very probable. For years she had lived in an atmosphere "infected" with tobacco smoke — her father, husband and son were all heavy smokers. Bosley found it "natural" that women who lived in rooms, especially those with windows closed during the winter season, in which the male family members smoked, would inhale tobacco smoke and acquire tobacco heart. Bosley had, of course, discussed in his piece the dangers and damage of passive smoking long before it was known and before it acquired that name.[37]

5

The Opposition, 1880–1908

"American womanhood and childhood must be rescued from the cigarette peril."
— Lucy Page Gaston, 1907

"Oh, the vile cigarette ... I feel outraged at being compelled to smell this poison in the street. I have the right to take cigars and cigarettes from men's mouths in self defense."
— Carry Nation, 1908

"[Reformer] Lucy [Page Gaston] never had a beau. Instead she had a call from God to warn the public, boys especially, against the evils of the cigarette."
— Frances Warfield, 1930

A strong opposition to women smoking in America quickly surfaced. It involved individuals acting alone using a range of tactics, from sermonizing and lecturing to more direct action, and organized groups with an anticigarette plank in their agenda or with such a position as the sole reason for the group's existence. Although the opposition usually was against smoking by anyone (male and female) often the fight limited its targeting to women and/or minors. Both genders were involved in the anti-smoking fight, but women took a lead role. The best-known reformer in that field was a woman. No comparable opposition movement existed in Europe. First though, females had to overcome the passiveness inculcated into them by society before they could agitate. An 1886 column with odds and ends of advice for wives offered the opinion that it was a wife's duty to make a man's home pleasant to him. If her husband smoked, she must not complain. Rather, "If he likes smoking let him have all he wants of it. The smoke will kill insects, the ashes will keep moths out of the carpet, and a little good-nature will teach a man to be as neat about his smoking as you would be about your tea."[1]

If women were at the forefront of the opposition, it was also due to societal values—women were moral and pure creatures with an ethical duty to lead the way in reform. Men were held to be on a lower moral plane than were women and in need of guidance in that area. An 1893 letter to the editor of the *Los Angeles Times* was about women never complaining about tobacco-smoking men blowing smoke in their faces (and into the faces of children) in public places and on conveyances. That letter writer urged women to organize and influence men away from tobacco, to press for legislation, and so on. He cited a Dr. Remondino of San Diego as arguing that a woman who allowed a man unrestricted liberty to smoke in her presence at all times and under all circumstances lost something. "Instead of creating in herself an ideal and setting upon herself her own price, she loses the power to make brutes men and men divine, and comes down from her God-given pedestal of purity and goodness to the level of the debased habits of men." Sadly noted by the letter writer were couples walking together in the parks and the streets "and mark how the female has learned to tolerate the smoking habits of her companion."[2]

Many women did come forward to fight the weed. It was just one of many moral wars then under way in America, including the temperance movement to abolish liquor and a women's rights movement that agitated for the vote for women. An example of the individual reformer was Myra McHenry of Wichita, Kansas, active in that state in the 1880s and 1890s. Next to drinking and gambling, smoking had been the most targeted vice in Kansas. Reformers were especially angered in 1881 when machine-made cigarettes were introduced. They were cheaper and more accessible than the roll-your-own type and much cheaper than cigars. Thus, women and children were more susceptible to the lure of the cigarette, or "the little white slaver" as reformers throughout America took to calling them. Temperance organizations began including antismoking messages in their campaigns in an effort to promote "clean living." McHenry was a reformer who fought for antismoking laws and for temperance and women's suffrage. She was jailed over 40 times, usually for blocking sidewalks and disturbing the peace. McHenry used the local newspapers to promote her views and lobbied the Kansas legislature to enact reform laws. As a result of her efforts, along with those of other reformers, Kansas became one of several states to pass anticigarette laws by 1890 — banning the sale of cigarettes to minors. (Reform groups usually failed then to get laws that banned the sale of cigarettes to all persons, but often won a compromise law — a prohibition on sales to minors.)[3]

A couple of years after that Kansas law went into effect, McHenry swore out a complaint for the arrest of Harris Stine, a 14-year-old boy, whom she charged with smoking, alleging he was puffing on a pipe while standing in the street, contrary to law, when McHenry spotted him. When accosted and lectured by her, the boy became "sassy," said the reformer, so the arrest warrant followed. Although laws against smoking in public by minors had been on both the state and city statute books for two years, the complaint against Stine was the first ever made in Wichita. City officials explained the reason for that was the law was hard to enforce in cities the size of Wichita, though they claimed it was well enforced in smaller Kansas towns. In larger centers, such as Wichita, were reported to be a large number of youths under 21 years of age who used tobacco. "I was one of the women who was instrumental in getting this law passed in the state legislature, and I propose to see that it is enforced in Wichita as well as in other cities in the state," declared McHenry. "Since my return to Wichita I have noticed that the authorities do not attempt to enforce the law, so I swore out the warrant in order to attract the citizens' attention."[4]

Mrs. Ballington Booth addressed a large crowd in 1895 at the Salvation Army headquarters in New York at a meeting conducted entirely by the women members of the organization. Part of her address was to attack the so-called new woman, the one who said she was trying to emancipate females—one "who has sacrileged all the ideas of wifehood and motherhood, who, by her coarse and brazen affectations; becomes rather worse than a mock-man," Booth complained. "She has an insane idea that she is emancipating her sisters.... We, the true new women, say, however, that we do not want her to emancipate us. For we are trying to raise men to a higher sphere and to be a helpmate to him, while she is trying to tread him under foot." Booth wanted to get rid of certain aspects of this new woman, especially her use of the weed.[5]

At the regular monthly meeting of the women's group Sorosis in New York in 1897, one of the speakers was Dr. Catherine G. Townsend, who warned against the use of narcotics she felt threatened home life — opium, cocaine, and tobacco. She said, "Tobacco is undoubtedly a depressing though agreeable poison. It is particularly injurious to persons of an emotional and oversensitive nervous system, and hence it would harm more women proportionally than it would men." As well, she thought tobacco use would shatter the nervous system and an inveterate smoker would become dyspeptic. Townsend added that she did not find much smoking among the women of the lower classes. "I have found a few of the younger women with whom I have had dealings who smoked," she explained. "But they were not representative types. They were the more frivolous girls who would smoke a cigarette or a cigar or anything that their friends would offer them."[6]

Carry Nation, a notorious reformer, was best remembered for her role in the campaign against alcohol, which succeeded in bringing Prohibition to America for over a decade. But Nation was outspoken as well on a number of other reform issues of the era, such as the vote for women, female dress, gambling, and smoking. All this was against a backdrop of the firm belief that human behavior could be corrected through persuasion and legislation. Tobacco was said to have earned Nation's wrath almost as much as alcohol. It was not unusual for her to approach a man on the street, pull a cigar out of his mouth, throw it to the ground and stomp on it. Nation told an interviewer in 1901 "[It is] the rudest thing ... a man throwing his smoke into the face of women and children as they pass up and down the street. Have you a right to throw in my mouth what you puff out of yours? That foul smoke and breath! And you would like to be called a gentleman."[7]

Circulated in 1904 was a story that Nation had placed a wager with anticigarette crusader Lucy Page Gaston over whether President Theodore Roosevelt smoked. Usually the story indicated that Nation lost the wager. Roosevelt, who suffered from asthma, apparently smoked a cigar as a child when it was believed doing so would help his condition. But that appeared to be his only experience with tobacco. According to Nation's version of the story, she was in Gaston's office (from where she presided as president of the National Anti-Cigarette League) in the spring of 1904 when she noticed a picture of Roosevelt on the wall. She asked Gaston if she was not aware that the man was a cigarette smoker. One thing led to another, and Nation told Gaston to write to Roosevelt and if he wrote back that he did not smoke cigarettes Nation would give Gaston $50 for her group's work. After Gaston wrote, Roosevelt's secretary, Mr. Loeb, replied that his employer did not use tobacco in any form and never had. But Nation would not accept that as proof, feeling it was a sham — a way to lie without actually lying — getting somebody else to write. (Nation had once been burned by that tactic by President William McKinley. Wanting to deny he rented a property he owned in Canton, Ohio, for saloon purposes, he got his minister to write the denial.) Because of that, Nation never paid Gaston the $50 but admitted the stories of the wager that circulated around America all claimed she lost the wager and paid up the $50.[8]

In her autobiography, *The Use and Need of the Life of Carry A. Nation,* she wrote, "Oh, the vile cigarette! What smell can be worse and more poisonous? I feel outraged at being compelled to smell this poison in the street. I have the right to take cigars and cigarettes from men's mouths in self-defense."[9]

Religious figures were also prominent in the opposition ranks. The Reverend Milton B. Williams of the First Methodist Episcopal Church of Oak Park (greater Chicago) gave a discourse in 1906 titled "The Latest Social Folly," in which he declared that women, with their cigarettes, wine and bridge whist were more than first cousins "to the swaggering racehorse sport or the man who makes a living by gambling." He worried the women of the wealthy classes were prey to influences that threatened their destruction because increasing numbers of women in the fashionable world were becoming addicted to cigarettes. "They are daily growing bolder in the matter of smoking in public. The non-smoking woman is said to be the exception in many fashionable restaurants and cafés and railway men say many women habitually smoke in their reserved compartments on long journeys," worried Williams. Admitting the craze was more pronounced in England than in America, he noted many in the United States were anxious to copy the European customs and were thus introducing and spreading the custom in America.[10]

For Williams, a subtle moral deterioration was then prevalent everywhere, especially in upper society. It was an occasion for alarm when anything threatened to lower the standard of womanhood, he argued. "For anything that degrades or cheapens womanhood strikes the human race at the cradle and in degrading the home strangles the hope of the nation." He concluded by wondering what could be done, moaning, "but what shall we say of the female creatures with a paper cigarette in their teeth, decorated with progressive euchre prizes and nursing a pug dog, whose whole aim in life seems to be the evasion of maternal responsibility and gratification of the gilded self of her butterfly life?"[11]

American Tobacco Company officials offered a donation of 3,000 cigarettes in 1899 to a women's group that was organizing a bazaar in Raleigh, North Carolina — the heart of tobacco country. The women refused to accept the gift, saying they could not countenance the sale or use of cigarettes in any way. According to Josephus Daniels, editor then of the *Raleigh News and Observer*, later a member of President Woodrow Wilson's Cabinet, "If anyone had indicated in that year, that any North Carolina lady would ever smoke what [were] popularly called 'coffin nails,' it would have been regarded as slander of the good women of the State."[12]

The highest profile organization involved in the opposition movement was the Woman's Christian Temperance Union (WCTU), a group best known for its work against alcohol in America. As this group and others got involved in the movement in the late 1800s, the cigarette was an unusual and stigmatized item, especially for women. Even as cigarette smoking became increasingly popular in the 1880s and 1890s, chiefly among men, there was widespread resistance to the practice. Smoking cigarettes was widely perceived to be a dirty habit; characteristic of single, urban men, and a disreputable form of tobacco consumption. Early public campaigns against the weed were often directed at boys, indicating the idea that women and girls might be experimenting with the cigarette was almost never publicly confronted. The temperance movement, which grew in strength in the last years of the 19th century, often included antismoking planks in its platform. Tobacco, like alcohol, was associated with idleness, immorality, and sin. Reformers then typically attacked the weed on both moral and health grounds. Women were widely viewed as the guardians of all moral things and, therefore, played a central role in the battle to stamp out cigarettes. Around this time the National Council for Women urged legislation banning sales of cigarettes to women.[13]

Tobacco was one of the items that separated the morally superior world of women from the earthy world of men. In her 1889 autobiography Frances Willard — a main force behind the WCTU — spoke to that idea when she called tobacco a "fleshly indulgence" that lured men away from the elevating society of women. Females who indulged in the habit sacrificed their moral superiority. Said Willard, "No man would ever be seen with a woman who had the faintest taint or tinge of tobacco about her ... it isn't thinkable." Willard's mother had used snuff.[14]

On a November afternoon in 1890, Mrs. Helen L. Bullock, the national organizer of the WCTU, addressed 42 small boys and 35 little girls in the Sunday school room of the Garfield Memorial Christian Church in Washington, D.C., on the cigarette habit. She told them in simple, yet "forceful" language of the harmful effects of cigarette smoking and how the habit was certain to destroy both mental and physical health. At the same church the evening before, Bullock addressed a crowd of adults attending a WCTU meeting on the subject, "Our Dangerous Inheritance." Referring to the American Indians she said that statues representing them were to be seen on every street, always holding out and offering to the passers-by "his accursed weed, tobacco." ("Cigar store Indians" were pervasive in the era, and for decades to come, with the phrase itself becoming part of the national lexicon.) Bullock blamed the Indian for teaching the white man the tobacco habit. Vividly she described the action of tobacco on the brain, nerves, stomach, and heart, producing what was called tobacco heart. Although she also spoke against the use of opium and morphine, she "was particularly severe in her condemnation of the deadly cigarette."[15]

Sometime in the 1890s the WCTU published Narcotics by E. B. Ingalls, a pamphlet that discussed the evils of numerous drugs, including tobacco, cocaine, ginger, hashish, and headache remedies. By 1890, under pressure from the WCTU and others, 26 states and territories had outlawed the sale of cigarettes to minors (mostly those laws did not ban the sale of other forms of tobacco, just cigarettes), with the maximum age of a minor in a particular state varying from 14 to 24 years. WCTU reformers petitioned the U.S. Congress in 1892 to prohibit the manufacture, importation and sale of cigarettes. While the Senate Committee on Epidemic Diseases agreed with the petitioners that cigarettes were a public health hazard, it found there was no federal authority to take any action — only the states had the authority to act and to legislate with respect to cigarettes. In 1893 the state of Washington banned the sale of cigarettes.[16]

Even fictional smokers came under fire from the WCTU. Those smoking and drinking heroines and heroes of modern novels had to go, declared the group. Work to do away with those fictional folk, which was to include the enforcement of laws then in existence as they related to purity in literature, was to begin at once, according to Mrs. Emilie D. Martin. She was the national and world superintendent of the Department of Work for Purity in Literature and Art of the WCTU, and New York County superintendent. It was through her latter position that Martin was to begin local work on the literature in libraries and reading rooms in New York City. "People do not realize that in 95 per cent of the reading matter published the cigarette and tobacco are represented as indispensable, and the bottle and the decanter are omnipresent."[17]

Over the years the WCTU lobbied legislatures all over North America in their efforts against the weed. Typical, perhaps, were the ones waged in Canada, first provincially and then federally. Between 1890 and 1914, the Dominion, provincial and local organizations of the WCTU, led Canada's first campaigns for antismoking laws. Those efforts led to the passage of several age-restriction laws at the provincial and federal levels, yet they were considered a defeat by most WCTU supporters. Quebec and Manitoba were the only two provinces that did not legislate age restrictions for smokers. Deciding around 1899 that age restriction legislation had proven worthless, the Dominion WCTU turned its efforts to obtaining legislation at the federal level that prohibited the manufacture, importation and sale of cigarettes to all Canadians, a trade restriction that fell under federal authority. For the good of the country, these reform-minded women argued, adult men would have to give up cigarettes. Only the cigarette, and not all tobacco products, was singled out for a ban. According to the WCTU, cigarettes were more dangerous and more addictive than other forms of tobacco, and the paper wrappers may have been tainted. Boys were the main targets of WCTU efforts, and when they started up with the tobacco habit they turned almost exclusively to cigarettes. Men usually smoked cigars and/or pipes, although cigarettes were quickly becoming more popular. Thus, the WCTU could argue their prohibition motion was harmless to men and perhaps not raise too much wrath from them. However, as cigarettes increased in popularity among men that possibility became less likely.[18]

When a WCTU cigarette-prohibition petition came before the Canadian House of Commons in April 1903, the group had some of its representatives in the gallery to watch. With no suffrage rights for women and with none of its members in Parliament the WCTU, despite all its lobbying, was still an outsider in the political process. Mortimer Davis, the president of the American Tobacco Company of Canada (Canada's largest cigarette manufacturer), wrote to a Canadian Cabinet member, reminding him of the large number of male voters who would be upset if cigarettes were outlawed, not to mention the fury that could be expected from 36,000 tobacco merchants and wholesalers in the country. During debates on smoking over the next five years, antiprohibitionists in Parliament argued that prohibition was a female invasion on the male sphere of politics, an insult to individual male liberty and an assault on male leisure activities. Some parliamentarians slammed the bills as interference by females in affairs they did not understand. Toronto MP E. B. Osler attacked women in general when he stated "there is more evil wrought among the youth of this country, by bad cooking than by the use of tobacco." Instead of lobbying, he felt, the women reformers should start teaching cooking classes for girls. More diplomatically, Canadian Prime Minister Wilfred Laurier suggested the WCTU females would be better of with educational campaigning, thus not questioning male freedoms, instead of pushing for prohibition legislation.[19]

Between 1903 and 1908, the WCTU succeeded in guiding four bills to prohibit cigarette sales into Parliament; all died procedural deaths but one. An amendment to the 1908 offering changed a prohibition bill to one that barred anyone under age 16 from buying tobacco or smoking in public. It passed by a vote of 61 to 51. However, the WCTU did not celebrate because the group itself had abandoned efforts at enacting age restriction laws as it had found all such previous successes to be only hollow victories. That is, wherever in North America was passed an age-restriction law on cigarettes or tobacco, enforcement ranged from nil to very close to it. As the Dominion WCTU prepared for yet another prohibition effort in 1914, the Quebec WCTU and the Montreal WCTU went so far as to decline to participate because, said provincial president Mary Sanderson, any antismoking legislative successes they had achieved had been "practically useless," and the organization would be better off spending its time, energy, and money on educational campaigns. That 1914 attempt also died a procedural death. Age-restriction laws it had succeeded in promoting and placing on the statute books in Canada remained in place, but were largely forgotten and not enforced until well into the future.[20]

Although she has been more or less forgotten today, undoubtedly the most prominent person in the anticigarette movement was Lucy Page Gaston. Next to Carry Nation she was the leading female reformer in America. Born in 1860, Gaston grew up in Illinois amid the growing agitation of the temperance movement. In the Gaston household, the spirit of reform was rampant, with all the Gastons described as upright, nonsmokers, total abstainers, and all imbued with a fire to make the rest of the world as good as they were. At the age of 13 Lucy was teaching Sunday school; at 16 she was a fully qualified schoolteacher. Journalist Frances Warfield explained sarcastically, "Lucy never had a beau. Instead she had a call from God to warn the public, boys especially, against the evils of the cigarette." She became convinced that many boys ended up in trouble with the law, in juvenile court, and in reformatories because of the cigarette habit. Smoking cigarettes drained the body of vitality and the mind of its keenness, shattered the nerves, and weakened willpower. Also, it led to drinking, delinquency, disease and vice and to petty larceny, divorce, insanity, and death. Everywhere, fumed Gaston, cigarettes menaced society. After 10 years of teaching school, Lucy could no longer contain her indignation; she resigned her job to devote herself to the war on drugs. From then on she was never anything except a full-time reformer. Even at that stage she was no stranger to activism. As a student at the State Normal School in Illinois she led raids—a popular tactic then, especially against saloons whereby the raiders trashed the place, putting the legally operating premises out of business, at least for a time — on saloons, gambling dens, and tobacco shops. Under the wing of the WCTU, Gaston worked on the editorial staff of the WCTU's official organ, picking up the skills of a journalist. By this time her family had moved nearer Chicago, to Harvey, Illinois, and, first editing a woman's edition of a local paper, and later assuming the managing editorship of a rival paper, she waged war on Harvey saloons.[21]

Author Meta Lander, in a book that railed against the weed, reported, that perhaps around the end of the 1880s or start of the 1890s, among the various departments of the WCTU was one for the promotion of Christian Citizenship, headed by Lucy Page Gaston of Harvey, Illinois. Lander related that Gaston was greatly interested in the anticigarette question and that was the third year she had introduced an anticigarette bill into the Illinois state legislature. In that endeavor she was said to have secured the cooperation of leading educators of the state, young people's societies, women's clubs, labor unions, and so on. All those bills were introduced under the auspices of the WCTU. In the *Christian Citizen*, a "wide awake" little paper of which she was the editor, Gaston vigorously advocated the anticigarette cause.[22]

But temperance work, according to Warfield, could not hold her even part of the time; her heart lay in redeeming the boy, not the man. "More to the point, temperance work was already too well generaled. A complete, high-pressure Heaven-guided organization in herself, Miss Gaston could not then, nor could she ever, endure working within organizations," argued Warfield. "She saw the anti-cigarette front relatively unguarded, save for a few sporadic W.C.T.U. Sunday School pledge-signings, and made for it pell-mell, armed only with her convictions and the Clean Life Pledge." Once in a while thereafter she would join with other women in worrying a saloon or bordello, but not that often. Although her own Clean Life Pledge included abstaining from alcohol, her efforts were almost totally dedicated to separating America from the cigarette.[23]

Through the 1890s, in Chicago-area churches and schools she lectured tirelessly on the evils of the cigarette, browbeating young men and urging their girlfriends to use their influence for good by not associating with boys who smoked. With her brother Edward Page Gaston regularly at her side, she began to haunt state legislatures, demanding prohibitive statutes. Gaston's tactics were to arouse public opinion, to secure wealthy and influential sponsors, and thereby force foot-dragging legislators to outlaw the cigarette, not only for minors (many states had already done so) but for everybody. The annual output of cigarettes in America had increased from 1 billion cigarettes to 2 billion between 1869 and 1890, which was just half of the cigar output. For women, a cigarette between the fingers was, of course, explained Warfield, "the smoldering symbol of the prostitute." While for men of the 1890s, the cigarette seemed "unsatisfactory and effeminate. Again, there might be something in all these rumors that the coffin nail was doped, that it was adulterated with sweepings, cigar snipes, and what not; that its smoke was alive with poisonous gases." Moreover, that was a pious generation used to legislating evil out of sight. All Gaston had to do, the reformer thought to herself, to be successful was to prove the cigarette sufficiently evil. And that was so obvious to her.[24]

Initially Gaston confined her efforts to the Chicago area, but in the late 1890s she branched out into neighboring states, addressing school and church assemblies — often those audiences were already primed by the thousands of antismoking tracts distributed by the WCTU — organizing girls' and boys' anticigarette groups and administering the Clean Life

Pledge en masse. Those who pledged were entitled to wear the Clean Life button. Once Gaston's lobbying produced some type of antitobacco measure on some jurisdiction's books, Lucy pressed for strict enforcement. Probably weary of being badgered by the reformer, the Chicago police chief finally deputized Gaston to arrest violators of a new antismoking law. Within 10 years she had been to court more than 600 times to prosecute tobacco dealers who sold their wares to children.[25]

After a number of years of patient efforts, her crusade really caught on. In the late 1890s, sponsored by Thomas Brennan of the Chicago Board of Education, she and a crew of recruited lecturers invaded Chicago schools and churches in earnest. Gaston urged her audiences to organize leagues against the cigarette. Such groups wore pins and badges, sang songs and marched in parades. Soon, leagues were being formed all over the Midwest. Her consistent campaigning in legislatures outside of Illinois began to bear fruit. Newspapers took up the issue; some were in favor, some opposed, but all provided her with publicity. Finally a group of businessmen helped her create the Chicago Anti-Cigarette League. Seventeen male trustees were selected to give her the necessary prestige and the group was incorporated locally in Chicago in 1899. In 1901, the organization became the National Anti-Cigarette League (an amalgamation of a reported several hundred anticigarette leagues claiming a combined membership of almost 300,000 members). Responding to a request from Canadian branches in 1911, the organization rechristened itself the Anti-Cigarette League of America.[26]

Aided by anticigarette drives in other cities and by the Federation of Young People's Societies, which helped tie outlying leagues into the national organization, Gaston's message spread. From her desk she edited *The Boy*, the league's monthly house-organ, which reviewed the field, reported legislative progress, and combined pep articles, sermons, anecdotes, children's features, lively dialogues between a cigarette and a bottle of whiskey, along with items from the press such as: "John Jones, aged 19, is very sick and at times acts very queer, caused by the excessive use of cigarettes. Denver *Post*," and "Elizabeth Scott, an inveterate cigarette smoker, jumped from a third-story window. Boston *Globe*." Lucy was also known to wander the dingier back streets of Chicago in search of boy smokers. Having found one, she would harangue him loudly until other boys collected. Then she tongue-lashed the lot of them. Pamphlets on the evils of the weed were handed out to the boys, but she refused to let any of them swear off cigarettes on the spot. They had to first report to the Anti-Cigarette League headquarters, memorize and sign the Clean Life Pledge ("I hereby pledge myself with the help of God to abstain from all intoxicating liquors as a beverage and from the use of tobacco in any form"), receive a Clean Life button, then they were saved. Through their nearest Sunday school boys could also join the league and get to wear its pin.[27]

Early in 1906 Gaston sent out the following open letter to the press from her Chicago League headquarters. "Cigarette smoking of American women is unfortunately no longer an open question.... It has been denied repeatedly by those jealous of the good name of American women that cigarette smoking prevails to any considerable extent among respectable classes," she said. Although Lucy agreed the right existed to men and women alike to indulge in the cigarette habit, she wondered, "Are we as a nation ready to face the fearful consequences of the widespread use of cigarettes by women? Let not the tempted young woman be deceived by the rosy setting forth by votaries of the habit already under its enthrallment, for there is a dark side to the picture which must not be ignored."[28]

By 1907 cigarette sales and/or manufacture had been prohibited in several states, including Wisconsin, Oklahoma, Nebraska, and Arkansas. Hearing that a bill forbidding cigarette manufacture was pending in Albany, Gaston went to New York, knowing it would be hard to make an impression in that state. She wrote to the swankier women's clubs—Sorosis, Colony Club, and so on—urging members to join her Lincoln Guards, confident that where upper-class women led, lower- and middle-class ones were sure to follow. In her letters she enclosed cards bearing pictures of Abraham Lincoln and, underneath, the Clean Life Pledge. The year-old Colony Club had such illustrious names on its membership rolls as Vanderbilt, Gould, Gerry, and so forth. Besides asking for pledges in her letters, Gaston offered to address the membership of the club, especially on the evil of cigarette smoking. In her note Lucy said she did not presume to say what men might do with propriety, but that she felt that "American womanhood and childhood must be rescued from the cigarette peril." No club took up her offer to lecture them; no legislation came out of Albany; New York clubwomen ignored her, but she was not discouraged. During her stay in New York City (she lodged at the Martha Washington Hotel) she wandered the streets, stopping whenever she saw boys smoking cigarettes and haranguing them mercilessly. "I would stop and tell them the baleful influence of the little things and in many instances I think I won over boys to my side. I saw a number of them throw away the things," she explained. When she left New York, she left behind a local organization she had set up. Gaston also distributed a number of pamphlets. One of them had in it the league songs. The league yell went as follows: "We have signed the pledge of freedom / On our honor bright; / We are anti-cigarettes; / We're the boys—all right!"[29]

In response to intense lobbying by Gaston, her supporters, and many others, almost every state considered some form of anticigarette legislation (over and above laws restricting the sale of cigarettes to minors; by 1900 some 26 states had passed laws banning such sales). Between 1893 and 1909, 14 states and 1 territory (Oklahoma) enacted laws banning the sale — and, in some cases, possession of cigarettes. Two other states, Tennessee and West Virginia, imposed prohibitive taxes. Such laws were supported not only by Gaston and her people but also by the cigar industry, rapidly losing out to the newer competitor. Washington passed the first anticigarette law in 1893, followed by North Dakota in 1895, Iowa in 1896, and Tennessee in 1897. Mostly those earliest laws were ignored until 1900, when the U.S. Supreme Court upheld the Tennessee statute. In that case a distributor was fined for buying cigarettes from a North Carolina factory and shipping them to his business in Tennessee. He challenged the law by arguing it infringed on Congress's authority to regulate interstate commerce. The Supreme Court of Tennessee rejected that claim in 1898 and upheld the law as a public health measure. Rejected by that court was even the idea that cigarettes were articles of commerce because, said the justices, "We think they are not because they are wholly noxious and deleterious to health. Their use is always harmful; never beneficial.... Beyond any question, their every tendency is toward the impairment of physical health and mental vigor." On appeal in 1900, the U.S. Supreme Court upheld the state law. That decision gave a great deal of impetus to the opponents of smoking.[30]

By 1901 anticigarette legislation was a major topic in state capitols across the nation; only Wyoming and Louisiana had paid no attention to the cigarette controversy. Pending legislation ranged from bans on sales to minors to a bill introduced in the Indiana legislature that would have banned public cigarette smoking by anyone with violators to be jailed, fined, and "disenfranchised and rendered incapable of holding any office of trust or profit." Successes continued with Wisconsin and Nebraska banning cigarette sales in 1905, while Indiana prohibited even their possession that same year. Two years later Arkansas and Illinois also banned cigarette sales, although the Illinois Supreme Court soon struck down the Illinois law on a technicality, a decision that prompted Gaston to initiate an unsuccessful campaign to allow the recall of state Supreme Court justices. Kansas, Washington (its first law had not held up), South Dakota, and Minnesota joined the cigarette sales prohibition ranks in 1909.

In many respects the late 1800s and the period up to around 1909 represented the golden age of the anticigarette movement. Cigarettes suffered somewhat during the early years of the campaign; between 1896 and 1901, after more than 30 years of constant growth, sales of cigarettes actually declined, reaching a low point of about 2 billion sold in 1901. However, sales rebounded and by 1906 they had neared their former high of 5 billion, in 1910 Americans smoked almost 8 billion; 35 billion in 1917. People liked cigarettes. They were cheap, easy to smoke and more suitable to city life than cigars or pipes. As men turned to them in greater numbers, the cigarette was losing its effeminate image while at the same time women were taking them up in ever increasing numbers.[31]

During this period women began to take up cigarette smoking to an extent never before reached, albeit still a tiny percentage of women were likely involved. Mostly the smoking that did occur took place covertly or at social gatherings of the upper class. Very little smoking by women took place in public areas, such as restaurants and hotel common areas, because almost all such establishments barred women from indulging. Men, of course, were free to smoke in all of these places. Some of these women who smoked at social gatherings may have done so only under peer pressure, or to appear to be keeping up with trends. That is, they may not have been smokers in the more usual sense of the word. Prior to 1880, even fewer women indulged, but the practice seemed to have been roughly spread among the classes evenly. From the 1880s to 1908, accounts made it appear that women cigarette smokers were all from the upper classes. Perhaps that was so, or the lower classes may have simply been ignored in media accounts. American women lagged behind women in other parts of the world both in the numbers indulging in the weed, and in the places where they smoked. However, U.S. women seemed bent on catching up. Also throughout this period the cigarette became more popular in general (it was cheap and convenient) as men turned toward it in greater numbers. The very negative image of the cigarette, relative to other tobacco products, began to undergo a rehabilitation in this period, although that was a process that would not be complete until the end of World War I.

Despite the small numbers of women indulging, the practice was significant enough to generate a loud, bellicose opposition, led by women, against smoking in general by everybody, but in particular against the cigarette. Zealous reformers succeeded in getting quite a bit of legislation passed, but those victories were all hollow as the reformers found next to no actual enforcement of those statutes taking place. Nonetheless they continued, swept along as a part of the other great reformist crusades of the time, alcohol prohibition and women's suffrage. While the singular development of the 1880 to 1908 period with respect to tobacco was the turning to cigarettes by women, a setting of the stage, the major development of the 1908–1919 period was the spread of the practice in America until the habit of smoking by women had a widespread acceptance in public places.

6

Abroad, 1908–1919

"Smoking among women in England is so ordinary a habit that it is difficult for English women to take seriously the American prejudice against it."
— *Washington Post*, 1910

"Cigarette smoking by women all over the world is so common now that few consider it worthy of comment."
— *Washington Post*, 1914

Europe continued to have more women smoking in more places than did the United States. Opposition to the practice was sparse and muted, relative to that found in America. Around 1908 the czarina of Russia had placed an imperial ban on smoking by the ladies of her court, and all women of nobility and of society who had entrée at court had been notified that the smell of tobacco would not be tolerated at her future receptions. Reportedly that order created much consternation because "a very large proportion of the ladies affected have for years been addicted to the use of tobacco."[1]

That same year the café of a popular London hotel took down its sign that read "Ladies May Smoke." The manager at the Waldorf hotel explained that although there had been a time when women thought it smart to smoke in public, in his view the idea had become less common. At any rate he insisted females were smoking less than in the past. "We do not object to their smoking after luncheon and dinner, but very few now take advantage of the permission," he elaborated. "We do not, however, permit ladies to smoke at tea time, and I may say that I offended a lady the other day by sending a request to her that she would dispense with her cigarette at tea." At the Savoy, the manager said smoking by women after dinner and luncheon was not forbidden.[2]

During the course of a speech at a meeting of the Army Temperance Association in London in 1913, Lord Methuen warned society against the increase of the habit of smoking among women. He argued that females did not have the same sense of proportion as men and that when a woman started smoking she did not know when to stop "but got a craving which she indulged from morning until night."[3]

Although an occasional discouraging word was said against the practice, most accounts simply noted the continuing increase in its prevalence. At a meeting of the American branch of the Lyceum Club in Paris in 1908, a discussion took place on the merits and demerits of the smoking room and of bridge playing. A few thought there was too much smoking and bridge playing, but that was not the opinion of the majority of the women in attendance, who had long resided in Paris. One member told a reporter from an American newspaper that Paris was no place for the puritanical notions prevalent in the smaller towns of the United States. Some sister members, newly arrived from America, were said to be shocked to find club members enjoying cigarettes or losing a week's allowance during a session of bridge. Both habits remained the norm at the club.[4]

Another 1908 article declared that as far as women in foreign lands were concerned, especially Latin nations, "smoking is so prevalent as to be quite common." In Mexico the female elite were described as "inveterate smokers," and a young Mexican woman would not hesitate to smoke a cigarette in a streetcar if she felt like it. In the homes of the cultured and wealthy, the woman of the house did not hesitate to join her family or her guests in a smoke after dinner or at any other time.[5]

One 1910 account stated: "Smoking among women in England is so ordinary a habit that it is difficult for English women to take seriously the American prejudice against it." Reportedly the practice of cigarette smoking by women had increased enormously among London women. Some attributed that increase to the number of women's clubs that had come into being and in which cigarettes were served with tea or sold whenever desired. According to a London cigarette dealer, strong Turkish and Russian cigarettes were exceedingly popular with females, while Egyptian and Virginians also enjoyed a strong vogue. The only cigarette that did not then sell well was the one originally manufactured for women — "a small, slender, mild, slightly perfumed variety." Any idea of expressing disapproval of the practice by socially prominent women or otherwise (Alice Roosevelt was then under heavy criticism in America for indulging) on the ground that they were setting a bad example seemed never to have occurred to the British public, thought the reporter. A few years earlier an effort had been made by one or two critics to use against Mrs. Asquith, wife of the prime

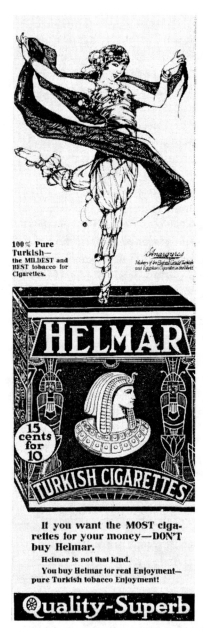

100% Pure
Turkish—
the MILDEST and
BEST tobacco for
Cigarettes.

Amargres
Makers of the Biggest Grade Turkish
and Egyptian Cigarettes in the World

HELMAR

15
cents
for
10

TURKISH CIGARETTES

If you want the MOST cigarettes for your money—DON'T
buy Helmar.
Helmar is not that kind.
You buy Helmar for real Enjoyment—
pure Turkish tobacco Enjoyment!

Quality-Superb

Turkish cigarettes enjoyed a
vogue in the 1910s, hence names
like "Helmar" and "Murad" and
what were supposedly Turkish
outfits on the models.

minister, the fact that she had been seen
smoking in a music hall, but England as a
whole "only smiled indulgently at her
unconventionality." At an open-air performance of Shakespeare, given at Lord
Saville's estate, Knole Park, Lady Mond,
wife of a prominent member of Parliament, "smoked diligently all afternoon,
and no one in the distinguished audience
present even glanced curiously at her."
Princess Patricia of Connaught, a royal
who was a favorite of the British public,
regularly smoked cigarettes after tea. Lady
Strachey, well-known philanthropist and
worker in the woman's suffrage movement, reportedly "smokes constantly without causing any comment among her
friends or enemies."[6]

One British royal not pleased was
Queen Mary, who gave notice that no
woman who smoked a cigarette could
come near her. Smoking was so common
among women in England then after meals
that one observer worried the queen's
order would involve serious deprivation if
it was enforced. Theoretically, it meant
that no cigarettes would be allowed to
females at any party Queen Mary attended — men, of course, could smoke at
will at such gatherings. A couple of years
later an account noted that if women
guests of Queen Mary felt a need for a cigarette, they had to indulge in one in their
bedrooms. Despite that a royal guest, the
duchess of Hohenberg, wife of Archduke
Francis Ferdinand, took out a cigar immediately after breakfast and smoked it.
Later, Queen Mary became a smoker.[7]

Alma Whitaker, a journalist for a U.S.
newspaper, reported in 1912 that in Russia all women smoked as a matter of

course and it was regarded as no more harmful an indulgence than consuming a cup of coffee. Much the same could be said of England, she added, where such prominent society women as Lady Alexander Paget, Lady Wilton, Mrs. George Cavendish-Bentlock, and Lady Maitland "are all inveterate smokers, to whom a cigarette is second nature." Also, many of the American aristocracy in England smoked, as did society women in areas as diverse as Persia, Turkey, Japan, and India.[8]

By 1914 one observer went so far as to declare, "Cigarette smoking by women all over the world is so common now that few consider it worthy of comment."[9]

Later that same year, cigarette smoking among women in London was described as a common and confirmed habit. The manager of a leading firm of cigarette manufacturers in Piccadilly said he had a large and increasing number of women clients on his order books. "Women smoke as a matter of course now," he explained. According to him women were more "luxurious" smokers than were men. They were then going in for elaborate cig-

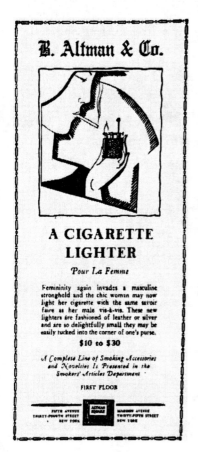

B. Altman & Co.

A CIGARETTE
LIGHTER

Pour La Femme

Femininity again invades a masculine stronghold and the chic woman may now light her cigarette with the same savoir faire as her male vis-à-vis. These new lighters are fashioned of leather or silver and are so delightfully small they may be easily tucked into the corner of one's purse.

$10 to $30

A Complete Line of Smoking Accessories and Novelties Is Presented in the Smokers' Articles Department

FIRST FLOOR

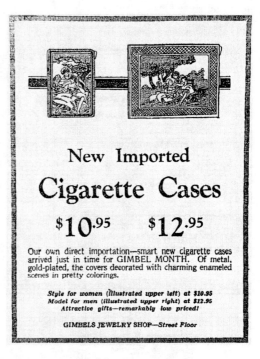

New Imported

Cigarette Cases

$10.95 $12.95

Our own direct importation—smart new cigarette cases arrived just in time for GIMBEL MONTH. Of metal, gold-plated, the covers decorated with charming enameled scenes in pretty colorings.

*Style for women (illustrated upper left) at $10.95
Model for men (illustrated upper right) at $12.95
Attractive gifts—remarkably low priced!*

GIMBELS JEWELRY SHOP—*Street Floor*

1926 ads for smoking accessories for women.

arette holders of amber and ivory, inlaid with gold, or studded with diamonds and other jewels. "And, of course, they have their gold and silver cigarette cases specially made to hold the particular size of cigarette they smoke, and charming little jeweled match boxes," said the tobacco dealer. Several London hotel managers, explained a journalist, unanimously agreed that for a woman not to smoke in their restaurants after lunch or dinner was then the exception while smoking with afternoon tea was not unusual. Said the manager of De Keyser's Hotel: "The cigarette habit is undoubtedly becoming general among women. The old social traditions and laws of etiquette are dying out. On the continent women have smoked for years, and it is from them that the women of this country have caught the habit." One of the more remarkable developments of the cigarette habit among women was said to be the teatime smoking in the cafés and tearooms formerly patronized by men.[10]

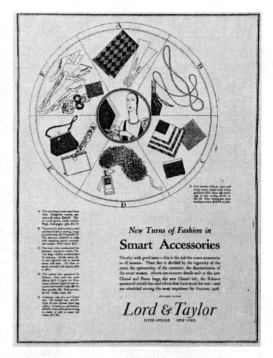

Two more 1926 ads for accessories, a sure sign the habit had caught on among women.

Midway through World War I it was noted that smoking after lunch was then permitted among the women workers in several of the most conservative government offices in London, and in other departments where official permission was lacking, systematic smoking among the women employees was met with a blind eye. In the offices of private firms and factories of all kinds in the city, the same conditions were said to exist. According to a London newspaper many women workers admitted smoking an average of 100 cigarettes weekly.[11]

A different 1917 account remarked on the dramatic increase in both the number of women smoking and in the quantity of cigarettes each one consumed. Prior to the war the women who "found consolation in the weed in sensible moderation," usually smoked from 15 to 20 cigarettes a week. But by 1917, the smoking "craze" had made so much headway among females that there were then thousands of women who thought nothing of smoking 100 or 150 cigarettes a week.[12]

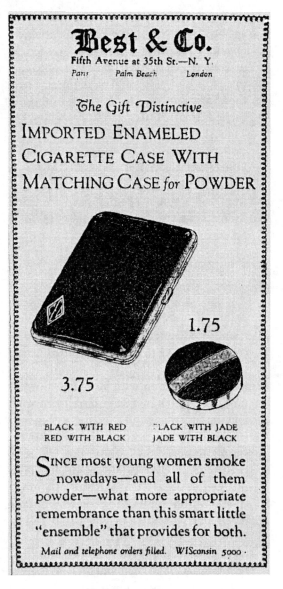

A 1927 ad for cases, which also proclaimed that most women then smoked. Accessory ads started to appear about a year before ads for cigarettes directly targeted women.

Late in 1917 reporter Marion Ryan wrote about a possible cigarette shortage looming and a potential need to ration cigarettes at home, so soldiers at the front could continue to receive their usual allotment. Should such a shortage become a reality, suggested men in general, then women should be the ones to reduce their consumption to keep the soldiers well supplied. All kinds of women then smoked in the United Kingdom, said Ryan, and they smoked in all kinds of places and at all times. They smoked in the theaters, in taxicabs, in streets at night, in clubs, in shops, in trains, and in bed. Girls of 16 carried "smart" little cigarette cases bought with their first war-work salaries while elderly women who had never smoked in their lives until a few years earlier puffed away "continuously at cigarettes, feeling much younger and a little pleasantly wicked as a result ...Women's clubrooms are viewed through a haze of blue-grey smoke." Many a moderate prewar smoker, observed Ryan, had become a chain smoker in wartime. With respect to any rationing, Ryan checked around but could not find a single woman ready to sacrifice her cigarettes for the fighting men to have her share, "But the smoking woman is on the warpath. In fact, I rather fancy she is stocking cigarettes, becoming a cigarette hoarder, for her excursions to tobacconists' have become more frequent."[13]

She said she talked to some 50 women but found none willing to reduce their consumption. One explained, about herself and her smoking friends, to Ryan, that they smoked on average 10 a day each. "Men, on the contrary, smoke from thirty to fifty cigarettes a day, I am certain. I should think if they were to halve the quantity they consume there would be plenty to go round, even with so many more women smokers." Another one rationalized that in a way, smoking by women was a saving. "It stops their longing for sweets and chocolates, thus saving the sugar supplies. All non-smokers munch chocolates or something sweet and soothing. Women are smoking more now because they are nervous, anxious and often over-tired. Tobacco is a help to them." Ryan remarked that many women were inclined to believe that the hint of a tobacco shortage was part of a conspiracy to put an end to women smoking. It would be a mistake, they believed, to give up a privilege they had won in wartime, the privilege of smoking practically when and where they liked. Such critics wanted proof that the outcry was really on behalf of the soldiers at the front. "And the proof will be if all men will give up their cigarettes or will cut down radically their consumption of tobacco."[14]

In another account the cigarette hoarder was declared the latest war development with both men and women buying as many as 500 and 1,000 cigarettes at a time, putting half of them away in storage. No sacrifices were said to have yet been made by female smokers; they were smoking as many per day as before and were buying just as many as ever, if not more. At a West End woman's club in London the secretary said more cigarettes had been sold within the previous two weeks than in the six prior weeks. A number of women confessed to the reporter to having bought "undue quantities" of cigarettes from different dealers recently to be well stocked in case of an emergency. Out of 15 females questioned by the reporter, not one had reduced her daily cigarette consumption in the past two weeks.[15]

By war's end, the British YWCA allowed women to smoke in its houses and Newnham College, Cambridge, made the same concession to women in pursuit of learning in 1919. The beginning of all that, thought a newspaper editorial, lay in the spread of smoking among British women war workers who found the habit offered considerable relief in the strain of hospital, munitions, or supply work. Having found it useful in war, they continued the habit in peacetime, and the British YWCA simply recognized a condition. However, a leader of the U.S. YWCA solemnly asserted, "never, never should it open its doors to the cigarette."[16]

7

America, 1908–1919

"Any woman who would express a frank preference for frequenting cafés where smoking is allowed evidences a tendency toward perverted, depraved states, and the ultimate end of such desires is physical, moral, and mental degradation."

— J. W. Nigh, 1911

"It's a burning shame that persons prominent socially should give parties in one of our leading hotels, and then by their example and encouragement degrade womanhood by smoking cigarettes."

— The Reverend Dr. Forest Dager, 1913

Among society people at Newport, Rhode Island (one of the most fashionable resort areas of the time for the upper class), during the summer season of 1907, the cigarette smoking custom among the younger women became the gossip of the cottage colony. Matrons entertaining were reported to be at their wits' end over just what action to take as hostesses as to when and where cigarettes were smoked during and after their dinner parties, and so on. "Before the season was half over the custom brought from Europe had become so popular that a woman smoking a cigarette was no longer an object of special notice," observed an account. "Women smoked at the cottages of their host and hostess and at their own cottages. Many of them had handsome amber holders which were carried in dainty, perfumed boxes," went a description. One of the leaders of the new custom was a well-known and well-placed society woman (unnamed) who was a guest at a dinner dance given by Mrs. Stuyvesant Fish in the 1907 season. After dinner she lit a cigarette and walked from the dining room across the hall into the music room and "enjoyed the smoke as much as the men guests did." Nevertheless, despite the habit's popularity, a reporter speculated the subject would arise in the upcoming 1908 season among women in the cottage colony who did not smoke. It was understood many of them objected to having their female guests smoke and might take a stand against it in the coming summer. "This is in keeping with the determination of the older set to make the season one of dignity, or, in short, to reform Newport by abolishing bizarre entertainment; so cigarettes will come under the ban too," reasoned an observer.[1]

In New York City in 1911, it was described as an ordinary sight to see women puffing away at private dinner parties and to see them "smoking occasionally in certain restaurants," but it was still unusual to see a female smoking in a taxicab. Still, the account said two women had been seen doing just that a day earlier going down Fifth Avenue in a cab from the Waldorf-Astoria. That the reporter felt it was newsworthy likely indicated how uncommon it was. Speculating, the piece wondered if it would become a fad for society women in their afternoon trip through Central Park to smoke when taking the air, in conveyances, "They may find it comforting and soothing, too, to smoke as they do their shopping." One indication of the continued spread of the habit was said to be the fact that almost every jewelry store in Fifth Avenue displayed in its windows cigarette cases for women.[2]

At a 1912 policewomen's convention at Portland, Oregon, it was said that cigarette smoking and liquor drinking were increasing among women and girls in Sacramento, California, and in Portland. Anne McCormick, head of the Sacramento policewomen, told attendees she had observed an increased number of intoxicated women who smoked the weed in the California capital. Lola G. Baldwin, head of the Portland department of public safety for women, told the conference she was sorry to have to admit the fact but her observations had convinced her the cigarette habit among local women, and especially among high school girls, had assumed such proportions as to amount to a "distinct menace to society."[3]

Around the same time female society leaders in Washington, D.C., were described as being divided on the issue of female smoking with strong sides for both the pro and con argument. Lady Alan Johnstone was said to have been a major cause of the division in Washington society circles by smoking in public and openly defending cigarette smoking by women. She had been seen "puffing at cigarettes while automobiling."[4]

Cigarette holders for women were said to be a fad among those with the habit. Mostly imported from London, some were extra long, ranging from five to seven inches, or longer. Available in numerous tobacco shops the holders came in different colors—amber was one of the more popular hues—and could be very expensive. One 7.5-inch-long model cost about $50.[5]

Another 1912 account stated that smoking among women was "unquestionably" on the increase in Washington, D.C. Evidence for that was said to be the sales of women's cigarette cases, match boxes, and other things such as the statement of Mrs. John Q. Thompson, wife of an assistant attorney general, that she smoked 60 cigarettes a day. "Many a society woman who regularly enjoys a cigarette in her boudoir read with interest Mrs. Thompson's remarks," said the piece. Among the ardent anti-smokers in Washington's fashionable set were Helen Taft, Mrs. Levi Z. Leiter, and Mrs. Walter Tuckerman. On the pro side were such luminaries as Mrs. Alan Johnstone, Mrs. Edward T. Stotesbury, and Mrs. Walter Brooks. The latter two placed on the habit their unmistakable stamp of approval at Stotesbury's dinner held a few evenings earlier in Philadelphia at the Ritz-Carlton Hotel, "when dainty weeds marked with the hostess' monogram were furnished to the ladies." According to this report the wives of many diplomats in Washington smoked and to them could be added many from residential areas "who are said to smoke at luncheons for women if not at large functions."[6]

Stotesbury's actions so incensed the Philadelphia chapter of the WCTU that it fired off letters to the society maven and to the Ritz-Carlton objecting to smoking by women guests. Letters were dispatched when the WCTU learned to its horror that women were at liberty to smoke in the hotel in general and that some of the women who had attended Stotesbury's dinner party had indeed smoked there.[7]

Even more furious by Stotesbury's actions was a local clergyman. Because the society leader permitted women to smoke at that dinner, the Reverend Dr. Forest Dager, pastor of St. Paul's Church (Philadelphia), was of the opinion that she and Mr. Stotesbury should be tarred and feathered, literally. In a sermon preached before a congregation of 1,000 people, Dager fulminated: "It is a burning shame that persons prominent socially should give parties in one of our leading hotels, and then by their example and encouragement degrade womanhood by smoking cigarettes. These people ought to be tarred and feathered. I refer to Mr. And Mrs. E. T. Stotesbury."[8]

E. E. Klauber, a "tobacco expert" with the Klauber-Wangeheim company, issued a report in December 1914 on tobacco consumption that year in Los Angeles and surrounding areas. Klauber said the people in that area smoked $30.5 million worth of tobacco in 1914; women consumed less than 1 percent of that amount. Women in the Los Angeles area were said to be among the most moderate tobacco users in America. Some 250 million cigars were smoked at an average cost of seven cents, while 1 billion cigarettes were consumed, at a cost of one cent each. (According to those numbers cigarette consumption was about one-third of the total, $10 million out of $30.5 million with cigars accounting for $17.5 million of the total.)[9]

Three months later an estimate of the number of smoking women there were in Chicago was made by Alice Clement and Mary Riley, policewomen in that city. After an investigation by them they declared that 5 percent of Chicago's women were cigarette smokers. In the Jewish, Polish and Italian districts of Chicago they found the percentage of smokers to be smaller, down to 2 percent. "We covered all parts of the city" in the investigation, said Clement.[10]

When New York newspaper the *Morning Telegraph* interviewed a tobacco dealer/merchant who had been in that business there for many years, the reporter was told, "Were it not for women the cigarette industry would go out of existence ... women and cigarettes have grown to be synonymous. Fully four times as many women as men are confirmed cigarette smokers" (all highly exaggerated statements). Women were good for the cigarette industry because they started the habit by taking up cigarettes, and staying with them, whereas young men also started with cigarettes, but regularly moved on to cigars. Behind the prevalence of the habit among women, felt the account, was the convenience of modern living. "Nowadays women have few duties and practically no housework, and no person can remain idle. Therefore they spend their leisure time in puffing cigarettes." As further proof that idleness was the cause, the reporter stated, "I have noticed whenever a woman becomes a mother, she drops cigarettes. She has so much to do then she can't take the time to smoke."[11]

Smoking by women in colleges would occupy center stage in America, but not until the 1920s. Prior to 1919 the topic was never mentioned, except when a prominent UK suffragette visited America to lecture and was housed in a woman's dorm room. The finding of numerous cigarette butts in the room occupied by Miss Ethel Arnold at Chadbourne Hall, the women's dormitory at the University of Wisconsin (Madison), when she was the guest of the university in March 1910 led to an admission on the part of Cora Stranahan Woodward, dean of women at the university, that the noted English suffragette was "a constant devotee of My Lady Nicotine." Woodward at first denied that Arnold was fond of cigarettes but when confronted with the butts she reluctantly admitted the charge. Coeds living at the hall corroborated the allegation, several of them having peeked through the keyhole to catch a glimpse of their noted visitor "complacently" smoking in her room.[12]

Noted American author Sherwood Anderson commented on women

smoking in his fictional classic *Winesburg, Ohio*, published in 1919. One story featured the Reverend Hartman, aged 40. One Sunday morning as he sat at his desk at home in the small community of Winesburg, he glanced next door and happened to see a woman lying in her bed and smoking a cigarette while she read a book. Hartman "was horror stricken at the thought of a woman smoking." When he began to think about her, he remembered she had been to Europe and had lived in New York City for two years. Then the clergyman began to remember that when he was a student at college and occasionally read novels, "good although some-what worldly women had smoked through the pages of a book that had once fallen into his hands."[13]

As World War I ended the use of cigarettes by women became an effective means of challenging social conventions, of deriding ideals of moral purity and the idea of women inhabiting a separate sphere. Smoking represented a culturally contentious, if not radical behavior for women. *Atlantic Monthly* in April 1916 said, "For a woman it is the symbol of eman-cipation, the temporary substitute for the ballot. Women smoke with ner-vous alertness." Women who smoked reported a newly found sociability associated with the behavior.[14]

Public Places

One public area that brought UK women smokers in contact with American customs at American shores were oceanliners. When the White Star liner *Adriatic* arrived in New York City in January 1908 from Southampton, England, two of the passengers it contained were Lady Juliet Duff, daughter of the fourth Earl of Lonsdale and the Honorable Violet Mary Vivian, sister of Baron Vivian and maid of honor to Queen Alexan-dra of England. They were said to be the first to startle some of their con-ventional American cousins by nonchalantly smoking cigarettes in the ship's lounge, where men and women were permitted to gather and indulge in tobacco in any form. An impressed reporter commented that Duff and Vivian "handled the cigarettes as if accustomed to them." Later they told the media they saw no reason why women should not smoke if they wished. Duff's husband, R. G. V. Duff, also on the liner, said his wife had as much right to smoke as he had. Some of the American women on the voyage had been smoking on the quiet only in their staterooms, but as soon as they saw the young English women openly indulging, they "went back and got their own packages, and soon there were eight or ten wreaths of vapor going up from the tables in the lounge." That took place a couple of days into the trip "and all kinds of cigarettes appeared between the lips of a dozen women — cigarettes with gold tips, silver tips, and plain tips, some monogrammed, and some not." Paradoxically, Juliet Duff declared she was opposed to women smoking in public.[15]

Also arriving at the port of New York on the same day was the Hamburg-American liner *Amerika*, from Hamburg, Germany, Southampton, England, and Cherbourg, France. Passengers included Mrs. O'Gorman — her husband Colonel O'Gorman was a retired British army officer and head of the O'Gorman family in Ireland — and Lady Alan Johnstone — wife of Sir Alan Johnstone, British Ambassador to Denmark. They both smoked after dinner in the Ritz-Carlton restaurant aboard the ship "and did not seem a bit put out" when, after the ship landed, reporters asked them if the story was true. Husbands of both women were on the trip and puffed on cigars while the women smoked cigarettes to keep them company. Each approved of his wife's smoking and, as Colonel O'Gorman remarked, "No Irish gentleman would object to a lady smoking."[16]

The activities of Duff and Vivian were the subject of several media articles, with their smoking said to have caused great excitement among American women on the ship who observed them and who, after they recovered from their initial shock, quickly followed the example of the titled English women. Duff remarked that although it was not the custom for women to smoke publicly in London, their right to do so on the Continent, in hotels and restaurants, had never been disputed.[17]

Passengers on the Japanese liner *Chiyo Maru* arriving April 7, 1913, in San Francisco included Lady Rowena Patterson, daughter of the late Earl of Huntington, and Mrs. Maurice Gifford, widow of the late Honourable Maurice Gifford. Both British noblewomen were decidedly against the suffrage movement. Patterson was puffing a cigarette when she opined it would be well for English suffragists to stay home and mind the children. Gifford, also a cigarette smoker, said, "It seems so bally strange to me that when American women come to England they find great solace in a cigarette, but when an English woman smokes a cigarette in America a big fuss is made about it." She added that she smoked on average 50 cigarettes a day "without any perceptible evil effect; in fact, cigarettes are a nerve strengthener to me." During that ocean voyage the pair smoked on deck or in the ladies' smoking room with complete freedom.[18]

Amy Lowell, a sister of Dr. Abbott Lawrence Lowell, president of Harvard University, and a well-known poet, arrived in New York City in 1913 on the Cunard liner *Laconia*. On her arrival she defended her actions in smoking on the trip across the Atlantic. Lowell described herself on general principles as a suffragette who firmly believed that women had all the rights and duties of men. "If I chose to smoke on the vessel I don't think it was anybody else's business," she argued. "The men were all smoking, and I would be false to my theories if I did not do so, merely to observe the conventions."[19]

A survey of the situation in Washington, D.C., restaurants and hotels in 1908, in the wake of the Duff and Vivian publicity, revealed that little headway was being made by women. Manager Haight of the New Willard refused to make a statement when asked if he would permit women to smoke in his establishment, but shook his head and "frowned severely." At the Raleigh Hotel, manager Talty said the question had never come up. Talty had a café and the rathskellar, in both of which men could smoke, but women had never attempted to do so, "and I am glad of it, for I would be compelled to put a stop to such a practice." He felt he could not allow anyone to behave in his hotel in such a manner as

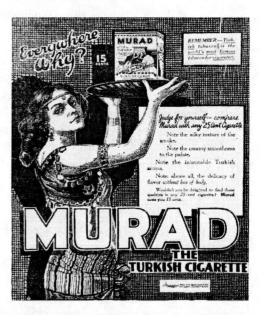

Left: Another very early example (1917) of a woman in one of these ads. Women in such ads formed only part of the background, but this female appeared to be about to kiss the smoking man, indirectly indicating her own desire to smoke, perhaps. *Above:* A 1916 ad with a woman as part of the background, unusual at that time.

to make themselves "unduly conspicuous. People should give some consideration to the general prejudices of others. I do not think that any of my women patrons would attempt to do such a thing. If a woman wishes to smoke, she should do so in her own room, where her action will not cause any comment." Duff's actions had not convinced Talty that it was the proper thing to do. "We endeavor to give our patrons all the conveniences and comforts, but we can allow nothing which will cause those who stay with us to condemn the management for laxity."[20]

Continuing with the survey, the journalist asked manager Devine of the Shoreham Hotel what he would do if a female tried to smoke in the public rooms. "I would stop it at once, at once," was the reply. "I disapprove of such a practice.... We have never been called upon to decide whether women may smoke in the Shoreham, but they cannot do it in the public rooms as long as I am the manager here." Miss Brown, managing secretary of the YWCA, was horrified by the thought. "Women smoke here? Certainly not. It would not be tolerated for one moment. We cannot allow a member to do anything which will call undue attention to her." Brown added that "smoking seems to me to detract from womanliness, and for that, among other reasons, I am down on it." She could not understand why anyone would want to smoke those "nasty" cigarettes simply because Duff or Vivian did so. "And in public! What has become of the old-time modesty of character and deportment," she wondered. "I can understand how some of those Eastern [foreign] people who have been raised to it can smoke, but I cannot comprehend a clean-minded woman wishing to do so."[21]

Three years later the situation in the nation's capital remained largely unchanged. "It has been settled that women are not to smoke in public in the Capital. Not that any Washington woman would think of smoking in a café. Certainly not," said a reporter. District of Columbia Corporation Counsel E. H. Thomas remarked that any restaurant proprietor had the right to forbid women smoking in his place of business, and if a woman insisted and persisted the owner had the right to ask her to leave his café. "I hardly think such a thing as force would be necessary," said Thomas, "because if a woman were to try to smoke, and should be requested to cease, she would hardly care to raise a scene of insistency." He believed public sentiment generally was opposed to women smoking in public.[22]

With regard to the city's more exclusive hotels and cafés, said the journalist, "if there is any first class restaurant here where women are permitted to smoke it could not be discovered" during his investigation. Most of the managers, though, admitted they had been put in the position of asking women to stop smoking. None, however, had encountered a woman who insisted on smoking despite requests to stop. J. W. Gibson, manger of the Café Republic, said female smokers were "absolutely tabooed" in both his grill room and main dining room. When the café was first opened a few women did light up cigarettes while eating, he acknowledged, but they all stopped when asked to do so. "No matter whether we personally object to women smoking or not, we must bow to public opinion and prohibit it," Gibson explained. "The Washington public would not stand for such a thing, and would quickly cease patronizing a place where women were allowed to smoke." Haight, manager of the New Willard, along with the acting manager of the Shoreham both said they preferred not to discuss the subject but stated that women who smoked in their cafés would be asked to stop, expressing the same sentiment was Levi Woodbury, proprietor of the St. James. "I hardly think a woman of any standing would attempt such a thing" as smoking in here, Woodbury added. Mrs. Clayton E. Emig, secretary of the Woman's Christian Union, said that public smoking by women would not be tolerated for a minute in Washington. "Women smoke in public in Washington," exclaimed Emig. "Well, I should think not. Public opinion here would stop it instantly." More extreme in his response was J. W. Nigh, at a meeting of the Secular League in the Pythian Temple in Washington. Describing smoking as the root of all evil he declared: "Any woman who would express a frank preference for frequenting cafés where smoking is allowed evidences a tendency toward perverted, depraved states, and the ultimate end of such desires is physical, moral, and mental degradation."[23]

Chicago's La Salle Hotel hosted a 1912 banquet given by the Chicago Medical Society to visiting German physicians and their wives. Well-known reformer and activist Jane Addams (a nonsmoker) was one of those present. A day later Mrs. Richard Mond, wife of one of Germany's eminent physicians, commented, "To be sure we smoked. Smoking by women in Germany is so common under such circumstances that we think nothing of it. I am rather sorry we ran counter to American customs, but the mere fact of smoking does not strike as unbecoming." Addams remarked she did not think it was very courteous to entertain foreign women and then criticize their customs. "The women who smoked at the banquet did so without any consciousness of breaking any custom. I am sure it never occurred to them that it would attract any undue publicity," she argued. "It is not the custom here, and an American woman who smokes breaks the customs and does so with full consciousness of her act."[24]

Countess Wolfgang of Germany was on a world tour with her husband that included a stop at the Hotel St. Regis in New York City in summer 1909. She grumbled that it was "absurd" Americans did not allow women to smoke in the hotels. "Such a privilege is not denied women in Europe. Oh, of course one may smoke in her own room, as the manager will politely tell you, but I mean in the dining rooms," Wolfgang elaborated. "What is there objectionable if a woman smokes her cigarette after meals at the table? In this respect the American women are not up to date." Additionally, she declared "In Germany we try to please our American and foreign travelers. I know that many American women smoke in public dining rooms when they are abroad, and it is surprising that they are not allowed to do the same at home."[25]

A party of four (two men and two women) entered the Ritz-Carlton Hotel in New York City in December 1910, just a few days after the new place opened to the public, and sat down at a table in the center of the big dining room. After the last course they had coffee, and one couple smoked cigarettes. Soon, said an account, "every diner in the big room had focused his or her eyes on the center table. The waiter hurried away to inform the headwaiter that a woman was smoking in the public dining room. The headwaiter called for the manager who came in, looked over the situation, and went back out. Nothing was said and the woman calmly finished her cigarette without interference." A reporter later called on Ritz-Carlton vice president Mr. Harris to determine the company's policy. "You see, I can't presume to teach American women anything at all. They know perfectly well what is right and what is wrong," Harris said. "So I have set no rules on the question of smoking. American women know best what is the correct thing to do in a public restaurant, and I would never dream of posing as an arbiter of etiquette." When the reporter asked Harris to clarify what he found to be a vague policy—could women smoke or not?—Harris simply repeated his earlier statement word for word.[26]

When the guests left the dining room at the Plaza hotel one night early in 1911 to take their coffee in the Palm Garden room and listen to the orchestra, a woman took out a gold-mounted cigarette holder and began to puff at a cigarette at the table with her escort. Her example, reportedly, was quickly followed by three other women lighting up. Soon the matter was reported to the manager, Mr. Skinner. He quickly sent a request to the four females to kindly discontinue smoking as that could not be allowed in the public rooms of the hotel. All four complied immediately.[27]

Later in 1911 George Considine, proprietor of New York's Metropole Hotel was resourceful in dealing with an awkward situation when an actress insisted on smoking in the dining room. She asserted she would smoke if she wanted to and dared him to throw her out. Summoning a waiter, Considine pointed to a large, seven-foot-high folding screen over in a corner. Under Considine's instructions the waiter entirely enclosed the woman and her table behind the screen; no one else in the dining room could see her. "The place is mine," Considine told the actress. "I can put a screen wherever I please. I please to place it around this table. Smoke as long as you like." About two minutes later the actress left the establishment.[28]

But inroads were being made here and there. At the end of 1910 the management of the Palace and Fairmont hotels in San Francisco had a one-year-old policy in place of granting women equal privilege with men as far as smoking was concerned. So satisfactory had been that experiment that the management had decided to continue it on a permanent basis and let females smoke as much as they pleased. Women could smoke in the great court of the Palace and in the lobbies, hallways, rooms, or anywhere else in the two large hotels. No restrictions were to be placed on the locations where women could smoke, nor on the format in which tobacco was consumed — that is, women could smoke cigarettes, cigars, pipes, and so on. Originally permission for women to smoke had been granted a year earlier at the time of the opening of the Palace Hotel. "It was forced by the action of a group of English women, wives of titled Britishers, who were at the Fairmont," explained a company spokesman. "They smoked in the dining room and in the lobbies, apparently oblivious to the surprised glances." Called on for a ruling, management decided that women would be allowed to smoke. However, according to employees of the hotels, "the habit of smoking has not increased during the past year among the women of San Francisco. Few instances of women smoking in even the grills have been observed."[29]

William Morris owned a number of vaudeville theaters throughout the United States. At a cost of $3 million he was building a new theater in Chicago in 1910 at the corner of Madison Street and Wabash Avenue. When it was announced that the building was to contain a smoking room for women, it was reported that "all Chicago gasped" and the news went across America.[30]

Hammerstein's Victoria Theatre (a vaudeville house in New York City) held a suffrage week in 1912. One participating group was the Woman's Political Union (WPU, an organization of suffragists), which had purple, green and white for their colors. Those were the colors of the English suffragettes and the WPU had adopted some of the English methods, and cigarette sales happened to be one of them. A number of packs were brought over from England a couple of years earlier by a prominent New York woman and the "Votes for Women" brand on the packs in purple, green and white caused them to all be sold quickly. Then someone with the WPU decided it would be a good idea to have some Votes for Women cigarettes made up and sold for the suffrage week, an idea apparently approved by the theater management. At the venue at least two WPU women wandered around selling the smokes, although not (it was said,) to small boys. Once again, they sold briskly. Then people complained to the press. Suddenly, the theater management denied it had ever given permission for WPU women to go up and down the aisles selling cigarettes. Mrs. James Lees Laidlaw of the Woman Suffrage Party remarked, "Votes for Women was a slogan which means purity of life, manners and morals," and she did not like to see it reduced to being a brand name for cigarettes.[31]

According to R. M. Haan, proprietor of the St. Regis Hotel in New York City, women would smoke in the lounges of the fashionable New York hotels in the coming winter of 1912–1913. He predicted New York women "will soon adopt the almost universal custom of European women — that of smoking cigarettes after dinner, or whenever they feel like it. This is a practice among women of the very best families in Europe." Haan added that the chief attraction about a modern hotel was its social side, and the custom of women smoking cigarettes had become so general abroad that it was impossible to prevent its adoption in New York. "It is a woman's right and her privilege to smoke," he said. "The custom will be general among women in the best hotels this winter, unless I am badly mistaken."[32]

Hot Springs, Virginia, was the location in 1912 where Mrs. Alexander Brown, "prominent in Baltimore society," set a precedent on October 13. While the lounge of the fashionable Homestead Hotel was crowded during a rainstorm, she walked up and down for half an hour, stopping here and there to talk with acquaintances, all the while smoking cigarettes. Reportedly she used an ivory cigarette holder, bound with gold, "a pretty little trinket that she waved around with the weed inserted by way of emphasizing her remarks." According to the account the ultra-fashionable had smoked there during the height of the season in the past, "but this is the first occasion when a woman of social prominence has been so public about it. The smoking generally occurs at night in the grill or card rooms."[33]

Many people occupying seats in the south Treasury stand were shocked by the actions of a party of men and women who were guests in Washington, D.C., of one of the assistant secretaries of the administration during the March 1913 inauguration ceremonies for President Woodrow Wilson. Apparently several of the women in the party were smoking cigarettes and drinking cocktails, "to the evident disgust of the people in the stand. Many unfavorable comments were heard concerning the actions of the parties."[34]

Near the end of 1913 in Albany, New York, Ethel Shackman of New

York City created something of a sensation by smoking a cigarette in the assembly chamber of the state legislature just before the session was called to order. She and some friends on the way to Niagara Falls had made a stop in Albany to see the legislature in action. While seated in the public gallery, Shackman lit up a smoke. First to see her was a page, who told a clerk, who told some assemblymen; then the visitor was spoken to. As described by a news account, "In an instant Miss Shackman was the center of attention. She didn't attempt any fancy stunts, blowing rings and the like, but just enjoyed her smoke and then threw the butt in the cuspidor. When it was all over the sergeant-at-arms of the assembly told her she couldn't smoke in the assembly." A puzzled Shackman said to that official, "But everybody else smoked." She expressed surprise at being told she was probably the first woman to ever smoke in the assembly chamber and laughed, "I'm not a suffragette, either."[35]

Cigarettes were placed on the contraband list at the county jail in Milwaukee in 1915 by

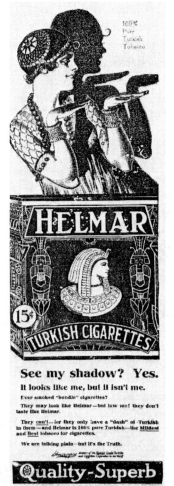

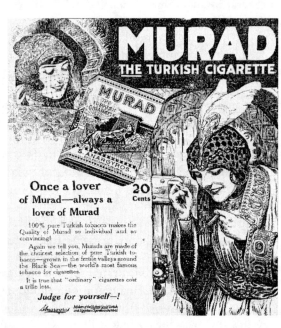

Left: 1919 advertisement. *Above:* Note the androgynous nature of the male figure on the right in this 1919 ad. Taken out of context, it could easily be taken for a female.

Sheriff Edward T. Meims. That rule did not apply to the men, only to the women housed at the facility. In previous years female inmates had been given the same privileges accorded male detainees— allowed to smoke — but the present sheriff was said to be of the firm opinion that "the air of the women's dormitory should be free from the fumes of tobacco smoke."[36]

Atlantic City, New Jersey, was the site of a new fad in June 1915, when several women smoked on the city's fashionable Oceanside boardwalk. They moved around in something called "a rolling chair" — apparently some sort of cart. Only one woman smoked the first day, but the next day there were several smoking in "a rolling chair procession" that was described as "blithely and seemingly oblivious of the shocked countenances of sedate boardwalk strollers" as they puffed contentedly away at their cigarettes. According to the reporter,

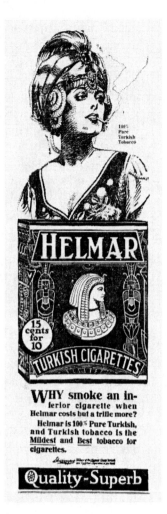

This 1919 ad appears to have been the first one that placed a cigarette in a woman's mouth. It was one of only about two that appeared anywhere prior to 1927.

> The sight of women smoking in public — so many of them, too— literally staggered visitors with fixed, staid ideas of conventionality. There were many indignant protests registered over the bizarre innovation, too; but since those who indulged in it were of apparent respectability and accompanied by male escorts, nothing could be done about it. The police simply winked, shrugged and otherwise demonstrated their helplessness.

Unnerved by what he had seen, the reporter concluded, "It was really a strange spectacle to watch handsomely gowned women, with unmistakable marks of breeding, rolling along the boardwalk in the comfortable chairs and leaving tiny wisps of smoke. They attracted more attention than the bathers."[37]

For what was said to be probably the first time in the history of Baltimore, females indulged in smoking at a semi-public banquet when they puffed their cigarettes in February 1917 at the dinner of the Maryland branch of the League to Enforce Peace, held at the Belvedere Hotel. Although that behavior was called a distinct breaking away from the old traditions of the city, the innovation was said to have attracted very little attention. The custom of women smoking in semi-public in Baltimore had generally been restricted to several local hotels, said the report, contradicting the assertion that the Belvedere incident was a first. Chief guest of the evening was former president William Taft. Toward the close of the dinner he left his table to greet one of the women well known as a suffragist. As he neared her table, she was in the process of smoking a cigarette. Suddenly she spied Taft coming toward her and rose. Somewhat embarrassedly she took a quick final puff and hastily dropped the butt on a plate, before reaching out her hand in greeting. It all caused Taft to smile.[38]

A lengthy survey article in the *New York Times* in March 1919 indicated just how much the situation with regard to women smoking in restaurants and hotels had changed. Earlier articles usually mentioned which establishments allowed the practice; this one mentioned the few places that barred it. From the long list of hotels in New York, went the piece, "few can be found where the managers forbid smoking" by females. Among the few, the majority fell into the category of family hotels, such as the Hotel St. Andrew or the Schuyler. In a few of them it was even the rule that men could not smoke at the dinner table, and it was readily understood in such places that the objection against smoking "would work with double force where women were concerned." The manager of the Woodstock Hotel prohibited smoking by women, not from a moral point of view he said, but from a business perspective. Such a policy paid because the hotel had a reputation of being ultra conservative, which meant it got repeat business from out-of-town families who wanted the conveniences of a Broadway hotel without subjecting themselves to any of the sights they might find objectionable. "People of that type would object to a woman's smoking in the same room with them, just as they would object to having a cabaret performance given at the hotel at which they were stopping," explained the manager. "Very well, then. We omit the cabaret, and we omit the smoking—for women." Asked why, then, the Woodstock permitted drinking, the manager argued that his patrons did not object to drinking; they did it at their dinner tables back home and "one cigarette smoked by a woman in our dining room would hurt the hotel more than any number of drinks."[39]

William P. Merritt, manager of the Martha Washington Hotel, declared the question to be a moral issue when he was surveyed as part of the article.

I hate to see women smoking. Apart from the moral reason, they really don't know how to smoke. One woman smoking one cigarette at a dinner table will stir up more smoke than a whole tableful of men smoking cigars. They don't seem to know what to do with the smoke. Neither do they know how to hold their cigarettes properly. They make a mess of the whole performance.

Merritt said also that he did not want the type of woman who smoked in public stopping at his hotel. "They can do it in their own rooms, of course. I can't stop them there, but where I can stop them I do.... If they must do it, let them do it where I can't see them. They can't do it in the hotel dining room." The Martha Washington Hotel did not maintain a bar. Also opposed to the practice was J. J. Lussier, owner of the Yates Hotel and the Lussier Restaurant. Declared Lussier, "I have always maintained that the old-fashioned type of American woman who does her own cooking and housekeeping is the woman who has made this country. Does she smoke? No. Are these new-fangled women doing anything toward the making of this nation? Not that I can see. All they have is a lot of wild, Bohemian ideas that never get them anywhere." Lussier added he did not want that kind at his establishment. If they came in and tried smoking, he stopped them. Noted in the article was the fact that managers of some of the larger and more conservative hotels said their old rules against smoking by females had fallen away "before the popular demand of their customers."[40]

Although large gains had been made in certain public places such as restaurants, if a woman went so far as to smoke in the street she still ran the risk of running afoul of the law. In fact, smoking by a woman was still used in court, sometimes successfully, as a mark against her to prove insanity, to get a divorce, as grounds to contest a will, and so on. Smoking a cigarette in the street, a young woman named Edna May was arrested at Ninth and Locust Streets in Philadelphia in May 1908. When she was taken to court the next morning, Magistrate Rooney gave the woman a choice of paying a fine of $6.50 or spending five days in jail. May asked to be put back in the cell for a bit while she thought it over.[41]

Betsy Hill, age 60, a self-described antiques dealer, arrived in New York City on August 28, 1909, on the American liner *Philadelphia* from Southampton, England. When the liner came alongside the pier, Hill was standing on the promenade deck smoking, an activity said to have attracted the attention of immigration inspectors. Also, she was reported to have smoked a cigarette while a customs officer inspected her luggage. She was then detained to be taken to Ellis Island for a sanity examination "on the ground that she smoked too many cigarettes," according to a news account.

When told she would have to go to Ellis, Hill was surprised and indignant. She argued there was nothing unusual about women smoking and some of the smartest women in various parts of Europe indulged in the practice. A reporter described her as follows: "Miss Hill was dressed in a neat tailor-made costume, and wore her hair cut short. She appeared to be a refined, well-educated woman."[42]

Two days later it was reported Hill had been released from detention after it had been verified she was one of Europe's authorities on antiques and after she had "demonstrated to the satisfaction of the immigration authorities that the smoking of a cigarette was not conclusive evidence of a woman's mental incapacity." Hill was released, wrote a journalist, "with a certificate that she is not only sane, but is a remarkably brilliant woman."[43]

Mrs. Maude White was sitting on a bench in a city park in Vancouver, Washington, puffing on a cigarette in the middle of a December 1912 day when police officers Jack Smith and Henry Burgh passed by and arrested her. When she appeared before Police Judge Shaw, he sentenced her to 30 days in the city jail for smoking a cigarette in the city park. (The actual charge was not stated in the account but was probably something along the lines of disturbing the peace.) Reportedly that was the first time a woman in that city had been arrested for such an offense.[44]

Mrs. Maude Arnold got into a taxi in New York City in August 1909 and told the driver to drive her around the city. He did so for 11 hours. When he asked for his fare of $20.30, she produced a nickel, all the money she had in her possession. She was arrested and arraigned at night court. Arnold said she thought she could raise the fare from friends and relatives and gave a list of names and addresses to the taxi driver, Isaac Utter, who went out and made the rounds. However, he raised no money and when he returned to court he gave Magistrate O'Connor a letter from Ella A. Powers, sister of Arnold. It said in part "I can only say that I believe if you were to send her where she could not smoke cigarettes for a short time she might wake up to the fact that they are her ruination." Powers also pleaded that Arnold not be sent to Bellevue, the notorious psychiatric facility. Arnold, though, was destined for the workhouse, unless somebody paid her fine. She declined to discuss her "alleged cigarette habit" with reporters.[45]

In the Supreme Court at White Plains, New York, before Justice Keough in 1913 testimony concerning the alleged incompetence of 61-year-old Susan A. Penfield of Mount Vernon, New York, was heard. Action to declare her incompetent had been brought by two of her brothers, who sought authority to manage her property, worth $80,000. Brother Thomas

D. Penfield instituted the proceedings. A third brother was fighting to prove his sister was sane. One piece of evidence came from Mabel Penfield (wife of Thomas), who testified that Susan resided at her home for three years and in that time she saw her smoke cigarettes and drink whiskey "almost incessantly."[46]

Wealthy socialite couple Sidney C. Love and Marjorie Burnes Love, part of the Newport scene and so on, engaged in a contentious divorce action in 1911. He charged her with smoking, among other cruelties, claiming he had no idea Marjorie was a smoker until after he married her. Marjorie admitted that she smoked cigarettes both before and after her marriage but claimed Sidney knew all along that she smoked. She said, for example, that while they were engaged she had asked him for a cigarette and that he had given her one. She went on to add that he had also encouraged her in the habit and never objected to her smoking, even offering her cigarettes in places where she thought it best not to smoke, saying that if a woman's husband had no objection then it was nobody's business whether she smoked. Marjorie denied she was an "inveterate smoker." She charged him with drunkenness, cruelty and adultery but not, apparently, with being a smoker.[47]

In a 1915 court case in Los Angeles Mr. and Mrs. Fred Shunko sued each other for divorce and custody of their two children. The lawyer for Fred asked him, "Does your wife smoke cigarettes?" But Judge Monroe disallowed the query and remarked that children would not be taken from women because they smoked cigarettes "in these times." Since women in higher walks of life smoked, Judge Monroe said he guessed women in lower walks might indulge in cigarettes if they wanted to. Fred's attorney commented that no lady could smoke cigarettes, but the court responded that was a matter of opinion. Mrs. Shunko was granted a decree on her cross-complaint charging Fred with "habitual intemperance." However, the children were removed from the custody of the parents, the court holding that both of them were unfit to have charge of them.[48]

Candace Wheeler, deceased, had her will contested by her father in Denver in 1913. She had disinherited her father in retaliation because her father had disinherited her. Attorneys for Mr. Wheeler attempted to prove that a Dr. Meyer had visited Candace at "improper" hours and that the two of them smoked cigarettes together, but the evidence was ruled inadmissible by Judge Perry of the district court. "Smoking is neither degrading nor improper on the part of a woman," declared Perry. "It has become a custom all over Europe for women to smoke, and the habit is spreading in this country. Men smoke and nothing is thought of it. Women have the same right, and they are not any more degraded by the habit than men."[49]

Medical Opinion

Medical opinion on the topic was mixed in this period. Dr. Rachel Skidetsky, described as one of the best-known women physicians in Philadelphia in 1908, spoke at a meeting of the Women's Club where she supported the right of women to smoke and that smoking "would undoubtedly be beneficial" to females if it were properly indulged in. She argued that men found relief from worry by smoking and "if a woman would sit down for five minutes before beginning her day and give the time to a cigarette she should be able to plan her day's work." And if she repeated that five minutes three times a day it would be "of much benefit to her." Many physicians held similar views, she said, but hesitated to advise their female patients to smoke because of a fear that what was offered as medicine might become a habitual indulgence.[50]

Not everybody agreed with Skidetsky's advice. An editor with the *Los Angeles Times* said he did not hesitate to say that to a majority of American women the smoking of a cigarette would seem equivalent on their part to taking a jump straight into hell.[51]

In offering reasons for the increase in women smokers a reporter in London argued that physicians had something to do with it because in prescribing for nervous women they often included a prescription of one or two cigarettes a day as part of the treatment. And so the habit continued until one found a woman smoking half a dozen cigarettes with her coffee after lunch.[52]

One medical opponent was Dr. W. A. Cundy, a prominent Pasadena, California, physician who spoke at a meeting where he decried the rapid spread of smoking among women. He said it was in the homes that cigarettes were smoked by women, and not just in the homes of the rich. Bizarrely, he suggested that cigarettes contained opium and young people in Pasadena who were unknowingly smoking them had contracted the opium habit but did not know it.[53]

During World War I attention was directed to the growth of the smoking habit among women in England by the report of the company physician of a large munitions factory that he had found 14 young women employees suffering from "smokers' heart." That physician worried because all 14 were potential mothers and their "children are likely to come into the world in a weak, weedy and rickety condition, paying the price for their mothers' devotion to tobacco."

Around the same time an army surgeon, who in the last days of 1914 declared that excessive smoking among boys was the cause of so many men proving unfit for general military service, had just stated that "one of the greatest evils produced by the war is the growth of the smoking habit in women."[54]

A different account from London in 1917 asserted that three years earlier a woman suffering from a smoker's heart was an anomaly but by 1917 it had become "quite a common" complaint. A well-known but unidentified physician estimated that nearly 10 percent of his female patients were suffering from illnesses brought on by excessive smoking. A worry expressed here also revolved around babies with a fear that a "race of weaklings" would be produced by such mothers. "It is the duty of every British girl who has her country's interest at heart to realize that excessive smoking might easily imperil the empire, and those who find 'the dainty cigarette' soothing to their nerves should smoke in moderation," concluded the piece. "An occasional cigarette is all right, but 350 cigarettes a week is bound to be harmful," warned the article.[55]

8

The Opposition, 1908–1919

"The sight of tobacco smoke issuing from a woman's fair lips is something incongruous with the man's ideal woman. It is an incongruity that shocks him."
— Washington Post, 1908

"I intensely dislike the cigarette-smoking habit for women ... no woman in our household ever has or ever will smoke."
— Mrs. Woodrow Wilson, 1912

"The time will come when cigarette smoking will be condemned by public sentiment and prohibited by law just as the use of opium is today."
— Lucy Page Gaston, c. 1913

As the prevalence of women smoking increased in this period, so did the opposition, becoming more vocal and visible, if not successful. More people weighed in with opinions, a few of them were even in favor of the habit. One of the earliest attacks in the period was on an individual, Alice Roosevelt Longworth, daughter of former president Theodore Roosevelt and wife of U.S. Congressman Nicholas Longworth. The alleged propensity of Longworth for cigarette smoking came in for caustic criticism in August 1909 from Mark Keppel, superintendent of schools at Los Angeles, in an address to the convention of state and county school superintendents. He declared her example had done more than any other thing to cause the spread of the cigarette habit in the United States and that example had a demoralizing effect on the women of America.[1]

Many more attacks were made on Longworth in the summer of 1910. The story that she smoked cigarettes reportedly set off a "lively debate" among well-known Pittsburgh clubwomen at a meeting of the Pittsburgh Playground Association Flower Committee (those in attendance were members of various civic groups). Said Mrs. J. H. Armstrong, "I look upon a woman who smokes cigarettes as I do one with bleached hair — with suspicion." Mrs. Minnie G. Roberts slammed Alice by declaring, "The higher the position a woman holds the more womanly she should be." A number of others thought Longworth ought to be ashamed of herself for setting such an example to the young women of the land.[2]

Just a few weeks later the four Christian Endeavor societies of Fairbury, Nebraska, voted unanimously that a public request be sent to Alice asking her to give up the cigarette habit. At the meeting it was observed that the influence of a former president's daughter would count a great deal with the younger generation in America. The resolution was the climax of a heated discussion on the topic in which society leaders in general who came out in favor of the habit were said to be "severely scored during the discussion."[3]

WCTU leaders in Minneapolis vigorously attacked Longworth when they declared she "is lacking in a womanly sense of responsibility, in yielding to a degenerate appetite and is aping the vices of foreign women, in showing her complete indifference to the moral teachings of her father, in smoking cigarettes ever since her marriage." Both Hennepin County and Minnesota state WCTU, organizations adopted resolutions on the matter, giving Longworth their opinions and urging her to discontinue the habit, at least in public. Rosette Hendrix, president of the Minnesota WCTU asserted that Alice had yielded to a "degenerate appetite" by acquiring the cigarette habit. Hendrix added, "A woman in her position, whose every act is chronicled by the press, should have sufficient womanliness to deny herself the strange delights of the use of nicotine in paper pipes."[4]

Members of the Cincinnati WCTU were also anxious to discourage Longworth. Sarah Siewers, president of the Walnut Hills WCTU, said her group would endorse the action recently taken by Lucy Page Gaston, president of the National Anti-Cigarette League, who directed that a committee visit Longworth or present a letter to her asking that she quit smoking cigarettes or publicly deny that she did so. Mrs. Emil Seidel, wife of the socialist mayor of Milwaukee, gave her opinion on the subject when she declared, "I certainly do not respect a woman who smokes. In my estimation a woman smoker is as bad as the woman who indulges in strong drink. I can think of nothing more degrading than such an action by a woman. The word 'woman' should not be applied to a person who smokes. She is not deserving of the name." After complaining that cigarettes were undermining the health of America's men and making weaklings of them she puffed, "Think then, what affect this same habit will have on a woman. Her duty is to be a mother, to bear our future Presidents, statesmen and citizens. Cigarette smoking by women means the ruin of our future generations."[5]

As the debate became more heated, more widespread, and public, and as the attacks on Alice became harsher, editorial writers weighed in, usually against the assaults on Longworth. Referring especially to the WCTU position, an editor with the *New York Times* called it "A form of tactlessness that seems to be peculiar to the sex so often credited — on rather dubious grounds— with possessing more than its share of that precious quality," as illustrated by its attacks on the ex-president's daughter. Granting that those critics had a right to their own opinion and a right to express that opinion generally and impersonally, the editor added, "But to pick out one woman who smokes— or who is said to smoke — and to make publicly an organized and concerted attack on her, with exhortations and condemnations, simply because she has a distinguished father, is both outrageous and impudent."[6]

On the other coast a *Los Angeles Times* editor argued the crusaders were not using a tactic that would lead to success in the case of Longworth, or in the case of any other woman of independent spirit, and there was the further question that even if such a course of action would lead to success, was it right to follow such a course? "Many things that many of us do are wrong, but they are included in rights which the individuals of the race never have surrendered," cautioned the editor. "Personal liberty in these matters that does not injure other members of society is a right and a privilege of inestimable value." Throughout the furor, Longworth and her husband remained above the fray. Neither issued any comment on the matter. The allegation that Alice smoked cigarettes remained just that; it was never conclusively proven, or admitted, that she was a cigarette user, during the entire heated controversy.[7]

Another furor, much briefer, over a single individual, arose in summer 1912 and involved Mrs. Ellen Wilson, wife of Woodrow. For the first time since Woodrow Wilson became the Democratic presidential candidate, Mrs. Wilson appeared publicly in his campaign on August 12, 1912. She attended in person her husband's daily conference with reporters, although prior to that she had made special requests that she not be quoted or written about in the papers. Ellen wished to have it fully understood that if she became the first lady of America she would not, as had been reported in a widely distributed interview, have packs of cigarettes in her personal desk at the White House and indulge in smoking them with her callers. Through her husband, Ellen asked that publicity be given to a letter she had written to the editor of the *State Journal* at Columbus, Ohio, repudiating an alleged interview with her in which she defended cigarette smoking by women. Copies of that interview had been mailed to her by citizens upset over the bad example it set. In that supposed interview one of the quotes attributed to Ellen was: "Certainly I agree with Mrs. [Gertrude] Atherton that any existing prejudice against women smoking is to the last silly and absurd. Smoking cigarettes is a question of manners, not morals. It promotes good fellowship."[8]

When the interview appeared in the *State Journal*, the editor of that newspaper was so incensed at the apologies for the cigarette habit attributed to Ellen that he wrote an editorial calling for the defeat of Wilson or a repudiation from his wife. "If there was no mistake about it," he wrote, referring to the interview, "Mrs. Woodrow Wilson shouldn't be mistress of the White House." When she appeared before the reporters, Ellen told them the interview was a complete fabrication and said, "I intensely dislike the cigarette smoking habit for women ... no woman in our household ever has or ever will smoke." Woodrow commented that though the interview was a complete invention he did not think it had been done maliciously, but attributed it to a somewhat well-known writer who styled herself Mrs. Wilson Woodrow, and hence the confusion. Reportedly Mrs. Wilson Woodrow was formerly married to a relative of Woodrow Wilson.[9]

In more general and wider opposition to the habit the *Washington Post* issued an editorial on the topic early in 1908. Acting as a catalyst for that opinion piece was the New Year's Eve celebration at Martin's restaurant in New York, wherein females were allowed to smoke in the place. It worried the editor that the fad was on the way to spreading to all ranks of society and soon women would be smoking in full view of the public in restaurants all over America. Grudgingly the editor acknowledged that morally and ethically a woman could smoke in public with the same ethical, moral and legal propriety as a man. Then he proceeded to point out why she could not, really. Nature had so constituted man that he of his own accord had brought himself to look on women as creatures a little higher than the angels. In the abstract ideal at least, "she is to him radiant, pure, and untainted by corrosive contact with certain of humanity's weaknesses," he explained. To all men, a woman was the embodiment of that ideal creature of his fancy, until she showed herself to him as something less.

> A glance may suffice for this revelation — a gesture even, or some more overt act. Now, in the sight of tobacco smoke issuing from a woman's fair lips is something incongruous with the man's ideal woman. It is an incongruity that shocks him. And no matter how much he may applaud it as cute, as proper, or as clever and right, a bit of the fine sentiment in him dies at the moment of the birth of the smoke rings.

Finally, concluded the editor, "Women may not believe it, but it is, indeed, true that no woman ever puffed a cigarette without losing some part of her delicate womanly bloom in the eyes of the loving masculine admirer who sat applauding it."[10]

Also in 1908, cigarette smoking by women was publicly denounced at New York's Waldorf Astoria where a social organization, the Gotham Club, met and discussed the issue of whether a lady should smoke in public. Mrs. Alfred Arthur Brooks said that in all the Bowery cafés and dance halls (lower-class clientele) they were putting a stop to women smoking, and "It seems a pity that places of the better class should welcome persons who can't even retain a footing in their own section of the city." Another speaker was Mrs. Imogene King, who remarked there were some women's clubs in New York that encouraged cigarette smoking by their members and that had rooms enticingly fitted out "to appeal to this degraded instinct, and I consider such demoralization a blot on our city's fair name." She wanted the Gotham Club to declare itself officially opposed to the increase of "such a crime" to "discourage in every way persons who attempt to corrupt our civilization." Later, another woman who had spoken against the habit confided to a reporter, "I often smoke, you know; but it would never do to admit it in public. The prestige of this club must be preserved."[11]

Carry Nation was in London in 1909. While traveling on a train, she became irate after seeing a cigarette advertisement and one for whiskey close to it, in the car. Unable to control herself, Nation aimed a blow at the cigarette ad with her umbrella, but the handle of the umbrella flew off and smashed through a carriage window. That caused the train to be delayed. Police arrived and took her name and address but allowed her to continue on her way. Addressing a meeting of women in London later that afternoon Nation observed that she had been in jail a great many times and had been beaten, whipped, and kicked, but she intended to continue to oppose "the great evils of drink and smoking." According to the account, "Earlier in the day Mrs. Nation took advantage of many opportunities of rebuking cigarette-smokers in the streets."[12]

Writing in 1909, journalist Lillian Bell, after noting a few examples of increased public smoking by women, wondered if European customs were to be introduced in America without protest. First she argued that nobody then was so stupid as to denounce female cigarette smoking as immoral or decadent or anything so absurd and out of true perspective. Everybody then knew, she continued, that to smoke or not to smoke was not a subject of ethics but a matter of taste only. Thus, Bell argued the real question was whether it was good form for American women to smoke in public. "The answer is, unhesitatingly, No!" she concluded. That many European women smoked did not excuse the habit among Americans, nor did it mean it should be imported. "Because we possess a standard of good taste which we claim is higher than that of any other nation in the world. We claim, also, a Puritan standard of morality which we consider cleaner than that of older nations." Why, then, she wondered, should Americans copy the habits "of peoples we proudly consider beneath us in morals and knowledge of what constitutes a standard of taste?" Any woman who smoked in public in America ran the same risk of being considered déclassé, as did the woman who painted her face too vividly. Bell believed people in America recognized examples of bad taste instantly and intuitively, "And smoking in public is one." If a female had to smoke, advised the reporter, she should do it privately, at home where it would neither shock nor offend. Bell concluded, "At present, however, it is still considered illbred and loose to do it publicly, and women of good taste would never make the mistake of laying themselves open to the criticism of those who hold themselves above any questionable practice publicly performed."[13]

Another opponent who subscribed to the fall from a pedestal idea was Dr. Madison Peters, self-described as a "famous preacher and author." He seemed to have some type of regular or semi-regular newspaper column, for the general title of his column was "Dr. Peters Talks with Women." On one particular day in December 1909, he talked to them about smoking. After noting the increase in female smoking and that it was then fashionable among many classes, he complained the "mannish woman" was undermining the social structure and destroying the sanctity of the American home. It was women's influence that shaped and drew out all that was good and noble in men and suppressed all that was bad and debasing. However, once a woman forfeited the respect of men she lost that influence, and her power for good was irrevocably gone. "The woman who smokes not only forfeits the respect of all right-thinking men, but she draws down upon herself a just condemnation and excites disgust," explained Peters. Woman was constructed along lines "radically different" from men, he added. "She has a more delicate organism and her nervous system is more finely strung, and is, therefore, more susceptible to the poisonous fumes of nicotine. A woman who indulges for any length of time in smoking inevitably becomes a nervous wreck." For Peters the holiest mission for women lay in motherhood, and the use of tobacco nullified that mission to a great extent. "The nerves are so unhinged and the potential vigor so sapped that degeneracy of the race follows. The woman smoker generally loses mental tone and power to concentrate the attention on any subject for an extended time." Peters noted that many European women smoked but that was no argument in favor of the practice, for there were many other habits among those women that American mothers would not dare to associate with the lives of themselves, their daughters and their friends.

A man might take out a woman who smoked for "a good time," thought Peters, but he would not marry her, and if he did, he would not stay married to her. "When woman, to whom we look instinctively for all that is sweet and good, falls below the standard man sets for her and believes to be hers, her influence for good is gone forever," concluded Peters. "If the sexes have to be equalized, I would rather it be done by refining the men rather than by vulgarizing the women."[14]

Miss Eleanor Sears, a socialite of some fame in 1910, was lavishly praised in print for being the foremost woman exponent of outdoor sports, a social favorite in her home base of Boston, and in California and Newport, a leader in every contest of skill that interested the upper class "and one of the fifteen really fashionable persons living in Boston." While not advocating the smoking of cigarettes, Sears was reported to believe their use by women did no great harm.[15]

Sears added that more women were smoking cigarettes than ever before and there was less objection to the practice in the social code. "Personally, I don't believe that moderate cigarette smoking could have any harmful effect upon the morals of the smoker." That caused several New York society women to respond. Said Mrs. Lillie Deveroux Blake, "I was brought up to believe that no lady ever smoked. I know many 'nice' women who are said to indulge in it but it seems to me that the practice is essentially unwomanly." Mrs. Clarence Burns, president of the Little Mothers' Aid Association, was more worried about the harm caused to a person's health from the weed. "Putting the moral issue aside, what is the sense in women taking up with a practice which men themselves have admitted is physically harmful?" Suffragist lawyer Mary Coleman said she agreed with Sears. She felt it was a question of personal preference and not one of public morals. Because it was likely very few men would declare that smoking was immoral for them, then it certainly wasn't immoral for women either, said Coleman. Mary Garrett Hay, described as one of the most conservative of New York's clubwomen, admitted she did not think it "wicked" for females to smoke. She said she would never do it herself but did not consider it morally wrong. It was a matter of taste and a question for each woman to settle for herself.[16]

The Reverend Cortland Myers, pastor of the Tremont Temple in Boston, charged in a 1911 sermon that Boston was being disgraced by a wave of crime, by gambling, by orgies of society people in leading hotels, and by women smoking cigarettes. Referring to a newspaper report that in the Back Bay area of the city tearooms were to be opened where women could smoke cigarettes, Myers puffed that the practice was a "very serious blight upon our morality."[17]

Dr. Charles Edward Locke of the First Methodist Episcopal Church in Los Angeles was another clergyman who answered the question of whether women should smoke, from the pulpit. Addressing his flock in 1912 he said: "There are some things to which one gets accustomed in men, which seem so utterly incongruous and vulgar and unwomanly in women, that every sense of propriety is violated and one of those things is smoking." Moving on to the pedestal imagery, Locke reasoned, "In a peculiar sense women are the high priestesses and custodians of noblest ethical ideals. Every normal man idealizes woman, and wants her to be spotless in her character and unblemished in her deeds. Any woman who smokes, I fear, is not very far away from the path of degeneracy."[18]

Well-known novelist Gertrude Atherton arrived in southern California on a speaking tour for the Democratic presidential ticket — Woodrow Wilson was the nominee. When her attention was drawn to criticisms of her from G. L. Robertson of Los Angeles, president of the Los Angeles Anti-Cigarette League, she said she would willingly cancel her speaking engagements if the people did not want her. "The cigarettes women smoke are not injurious. In the old world the women have smoked such cigarettes for centuries without injurious results," said Atherton.[19]

Alma Whitaker, a regular columnist with the *Los Angeles Times*, interviewed Atherton in 1917 and recalled the literary figure smoked her cigarettes skewered on the end of a long hatpin to save her fingers from the stain. Atherton asked Whitaker if the latter was "public." Unable to respond because she was confused by the question Atherton laughingly explained that she had promised the WCTU that she would not smoke a cigarette "in public." But she felt a soothing cigarette was essential to a newspaper interview and idly wondered if the interview process with a reporter could be considered as being "in public."[20]

When the editor of the *New York Times* raised objections to the practice in 1913, he raised a point that had not been mentioned before — an economic objection. The use of tobacco by the men already absorbed too large a part of the family income to warrant any further drain, he argued. If the women had to smoke he advised them to refrain from indulging until the economic circumstances of the nation improved somewhat.[21]

For Claude Cherys, writing in 1913, society was then passing through a period of unrest and uncertainty with the old order changing, but the new order was not giving complete satisfaction. One of the major problems he saw in society then was, in all too many cases, a lack of "cultivated taste." Cherys said he was prompted to comment after sitting in the lounge of a large, fashionable Paris hotel and watching women come and go in the public rooms. What concerned him the most was the "up-to-date woman or girl who insisted on her 'rights' and who boldly smokes in the public rooms of restaurants or hotels." Then Cherys issued the standard disclaimer in which he stated he had not the slightest objection to women smoking cigarettes if they wanted to—that he had many female friends who did so, but they did not smoke in public. A cigarette smoked privately was one thing, he argued, but the same cigarette smoked in the public rooms of restaurants and hotels was another thing. "The latter is an offense against good taste," he declared. Going on, he described two English women he had seen in Paris who "ostentatiously" smoked cigarettes. It was even true that "one of them was lying back on a lounge with her knees crossed in true mannish style." Cherys concluded that if a woman really enjoyed a cigarette she would smoke it only in private, alone or with friends; "Any woman who imagines that she is asserting her 'rights' by smoking in public is mistaken. 'Rights' are bigger things than cigarettes, or even cigars."[22]

At a reception given by the ladies of Mount Pleasant Congregational Church in Washington, D.C., for the members of the YWCA at the end of 1913, the Reverend Clarence A. Vincent made a sweeping indictment against what he termed the growing tendency to irreligion among the women of the United States. In particular, he singled out for criticism the increasing prevalence of American women smoking cigarettes along with the wearing of "ultra modern types of gowns," due in large measure, he felt, to the examples of women who had come to this country from Europe.[23]

Eugene Brown, a Los Angeles newspaper columnist, grumbled that women had recently been encouraged to vote, "play poker and climb trees," but now the last barrier of sex had been broken down because "the swagger hotels of the purse-puffed plutocrats have announced that hereafter women — meaning perfect ladies— may smoke wherever they please."[24]

Dr. William H. Allen, former director of the Bureau of Municipal Research and director of the Institute for Public Service, issued a bulletin in 1916 in which he set forth cigarette smoking among women and children as one of several alleged evils demanding correction. It was his contention that the whole fabric of the various movements for civic betterment in New York was being undermined by cigarette smoking women. "Think," fumed the bulletin, "of contributing charitable funds to promote woman's equal rights to smoke cigarettes!" Allen noted New York spent millions of dollars in charitable work but wondered, "What good does it do if the women engaged in it are cigarette smokers? The women who wield a strong influence in promoting uplift movements and who have the 'ear' of the city administration are, almost without exception, smokers."[25]

One outspoken proponent for female smoking was newspaper columnist Alma Whitaker. Noting in 1912 how many women smoked in other countries, she wondered why American women "should be denied this harmless, peaceful sort of pastime? For the life of me I can see nothing disreputable in smoking, unless it is carried to excess." Exclaiming she had never heard a really good argument against smoking for women, Whitaker waxed poetically that a good cigarette "is a dainty enough article — symmetrical, clean, innocent. Smoke is graceful, wholesome, soothing." A smoker herself, Whitaker came out in favor of moderate smoking both for men and women, explaining, "Many a murder could be avoided if the angered one would pause and smoke. Many a catty wife, many a bearish husband would become more endurable could they but be persuaded to indulge in an occasional smoke — the mere act of smoking makes for companionable feeling, for gentleness, for placidity." Apparently unable to contain himself, the paper's editor added a one-word comment at the end of her article — "Huh!"[26]

Whitaker returned with another opinion piece in favor of female smoking in 1916. Observing that William Allen White declared that women who smoked cigarettes were unfit to be mothers, Alma added, sarcastically, that many women smoked in foreign countries and U.S. females had been condemned for wearing short skirts, corsets, working in factories, riding bicycles, and so on, and in every case condemned as unfit. This time around the item focused on was cigarettes. Pointing out the existence of unfair discrimination Whitaker said no one declared a man to be unfit to be a father "for anything short of cardinal crime." There were all sorts of smoking males in the world, she argued, whose laurels depended on clear minds and personal fitness "who smoke like young chimneys day in and day out, but no one ever tells them they are unfit to grace their positions because they smoke." Added Alma ironically, "But, you will understand, it is quite impossible for a woman to run her home decently and bring up her children properly if she smokes a quarter's worth of cigarettes occasionally — the brazen hussy!"[27]

Alma's next prosmoking column appeared later in 1916 when she mocked the idea that cigarettes for women were instruments of the devil. "We all know when the villainess appears on the screen at the movies, because she is designated with a wicked cigarette which she puffs with horrid enjoyment. The nasty minx." According to Whitaker, 75 percent of British women smoked, and it was women who Lloyd George declared had saved England in her hour of peril by their loyalty, industry, and so on; to which Whitaker's sarcastic rejoinder was "must be a lot of unspeakable hussies. It is a jolly shame that any decent country should have to be saved by hussies." For Alma, the habit was no vice. She mentioned all the decent women she knew who were smokers and came from a variety of back-grounds—female physicians, doctors' wives, sportswomen, and so forth. "See them, after a round of golf or an exciting tennis set at the country clubs, produce their shameless silver cigarette cases and settle down to a cozy conversational cigarette," she wrote.[28]

At the annual convention of the National WCTU in 1910 in Balti-more, the keynote address was delivered by the group's president, Lillian M. Stevens, who stated there was no increase in the numbers of women smoking and drinking and that there were few female smokers. "I am glad that the national and world's W.C.T.U. has a department of antinarcotics," she continued, "and I am happy in believing that the number of women who smoke cigarettes in elegant homes or who smoke tobacco in any form in the tramp lodging houses are very few in this country."[29]

Several years later, the Los Angeles WCTU held its annual meeting at which it carried out the usual business of such a meeting — the election of officers, the reading of reports from various officers, and so on. Mrs. M. W. Law, the president of the group, read the president's report for the year showing she had made 177 addresses and had spoken 47 times at parent-teacher associations and 21 times before missionary societies. The treasurer reported a balance of $83 in the bank. Mrs. Milligan gave a talk at that meeting on the "cigarette evil" and a committee was appointed to confer with her regarding the establishment of a clinic for treatment of victims of this habit.[30]

Lucy Page Gaston and her organization also remained active among the opponents of the weed. James J. Jeffreys, field secretary of the Anti-Cigarette League, delivered an address in Washington, D.C., in 1911 before about 500 members of the Christian Endeavor Society at the Berwyn Pres-byterian Church. Moved by the vivid pictures of the evils of the tobacco habit 200 young women, members of the society, pledged themselves at that meeting to forswear the society of all young men who used tobacco. "My dear girls," said Jeffreys, "it is for you and others like you to reform the young men who think it manly to use the weed. You can do more than I can to fight this evil, and I call upon you to do it." When one of these new recruits in the war found a young man who used weed, she was urged by Jeffreys to "make him cut it out, or cut his acquaintance." Following his address Jeffreys descended from the platform and was surrounded by scores of young women. Each agreed that until her young men friends resigned themselves to the simple tobacco-free life she would forsake them.[31]

A clinic for women smokers was established in March 1914 in Chicago by the Anti-Cigarette League, using a method said to have been successful in breaking boys of the habit who had appeared in juvenile court. The treatment was simply spraying the throat with a solution of nitrate of silver. League president Gaston said 15 females had already been successfully treated. "Our first feminine applicant was a chorus girl, who began puffing cigarettes in a spirit of bravado," she added. Gaston explained the clinic was opened in the belief there were thousands of females in Chicago who would rid themselves of the "vice" if they had the opportunity.[32]

During the spring of 1915 Jennie Hobson Milligan, superintendent of the New York State Anti-Cigarette League, conducted a lecture tour in New York State and several Southern states, including North Carolina, Florida, and Virginia, lecturing to schools, colleges, YMCAs, churches and Sunday schools in connection with the national and state work of the league. Her purpose was to arouse a sentiment strong enough to secure legislation prohibiting the sale of cigarettes in the United States. At that time, she indicated, several states had passed such legislation. To accomplish prohibition of the cigarette, Milligan believed the ballot for women would be of great benefit. Mothers had shown that they would sacrifice anything for their children, she explained. "If mothers could get the ballot the road to abolition of such things as drug-forming materials, of which tobacco is one, would be studied and better understood, and then mothers would use their power in passing laws to abolish them. Therefore I am much interested in woman suffrage," she declared.[33]

Gaston blamed the tobacco industry lobby when by 1911 Illinois had twice passed anticigarette bills only to have them pronounced invalid by the state Supreme Court. "But some day we shall win," she declared. "The time will come when cigarette smoking will be condemned by public sentiment and prohibited by law just as the use of opium is today." Directly or indirectly through her efforts, anticigarette laws had been passed in some 11 states by 1913. However, as Gaston herself admitted, smoking went on as usual in those states. Tobacco manufacturers sent cigarettes through the mail; retail dealers sold matches for 20 cents or so and gave cigarettes away. When World War I came and the cigarette had its image rehabilitated, it soon became a patriotic duty to send cigarettes to the U.S. forces overseas. Nonetheless, Gaston fought on. She instituted legal proceedings against the patriotic organizations of Kansas for sending cartons of smokes to the front when, under a state law, cigarettes could not legally be bought or sold within the state. Gaston was unsuccessful in those proceedings, and the few people who paid her any heed did so only to sharply question her love of country.[34]

At the beginning of 1908, a resolution was introduced in the New York City Board of Aldermen by Alderman Timothy Sullivan; the resolution would have prohibited the use of tobacco in public places by women. With respect to Sullivan's motivation, a *New York Times* editorial stated, "He does not like to see women smoking, and he believes that the sight of a woman puffing a cigarette tends to weaken the respect men ought to feel for women."[35]

After a brief hearing on January 20, the Committee on Laws of the Board of Aldermen unanimously approved the Sullivan antismoking ordinance. It meant that if it passed the board it would be against the law for a hotel or restaurant proprietor or anyone else managing or owning a "public place" to allow women to smoke in public. Under the Sullivan ordinance it was not an offense for a woman to smoke in public, but it was an offense for the manager or proprietor of a public place to allow her to smoke therein, and for doing so he could suffer the revocation of his business license and also be fined or jailed. Impetus for that ordinance was said to have been the announcement just before the previous New Year's Eve that Martin's would allow females to smoke in its restaurant — an announcement that did not sit well with Sullivan. At the January hearing were 11 women and 15 men with 4 people speaking against the proposal. One speaker was Sullivan himself, who declared he had never seen women smoking in public places in his district and who stated emphatically that several leading restaurant owners had approved of the ordinance.[36]

On the night of January 21, the Board of Aldermen passed the Sullivan ordinance by a vote of 73 to 0. It went into effect immediately. Section 1 of the act said, "No person, firm or partnership corporation, or association, of whatever character, owning or controlling either as proprietor, or manager, any hotel, restaurant, place of public entertainment, or other place of public resort, in the City of New York, ... shall allow any female to smoke [therein], ... and an act being construed as in contravention of the provisions of Subdivision 14 of Section 49 of the Greater New York charter." Under Section 2: "Any violation of the provisions of this ordinance, upon conviction thereof, before a City Magistrate, shall be punishable by a fine of not less than $5 nor more than $25, or by imprisonment in the city prison, or by both, but no such imprisonment, however, shall exceed a term of ten days." Under Section 3, "This ordinance shall take effect immediately."[37]

Two days later, policeman Stern ran across the Bowery at Division Street after he had observed a woman take a cigarette out of a package and light up in the street. "Madam, you mustn't," said Stern. "What would Alderman Sullivan say?" At night court Katie Mulcahey complained to Magistrate Kernochan, "I've got as much right to smoke as you have. I never heard of this new law, and I don't want to hear about it. No man shall dictate to me." Kernochan fined her $5, and in default of paying she went to jail. All this happened — the arrest, conviction, and imposition of a fine — even though Mulcahey was obviously not in violation of the Sullivan ordinance.[38]

New York City Mayor McClellan vetoed Sullivan's ordinance early in February after he sent a communication to the Board of Aldermen in which he stated he knew of no provision of law that gave the Board of Aldermen the power to enact an ordinance of that kind. When the veto was exercised Sullivan was away in Hot Springs, Arkansas, and it was felt that nothing further would be done with the ordinance — that it would be left for dead.[39]

At that time the Irish political machine was a dominant force in New York City politics, with two of its prominent members both named Tim Sullivan; they were cousins. Little Tim was the Alderman and Big Tim had been a member of the U.S. Congress and of the state legislative assembly, but apparently held no elective office in early 1908. Neither of them smoked, chewed or drank and their political views were said by observers to be identical. After the veto was exercised a reporter interviewed Big Tim on the subject (Little Tim was still in Arkansas) at one of the Sullivan headquarters, the Occidental Hotel on the Bowery. Big Tim said Little Tim had been badly misjudged in the matter, as the latter did not sit around thinking up ways to curtail the privileges of women, as some critics had suggested. After Little Tim saw the ad in the paper for Martin's and had his ire aroused, explained Big Tim, the pair had a meeting and agreed the practice of women smoking in public was not acceptable, because womankind was "too sacred" to them. Big Tim observed that his own sensibilities had been shocked in the previous summer (1907) during a trip to London, England where he saw several women smoking in restaurants. He went on to say that neither of them wanted to interfere with anybody's liberty — "We're both great on personal liberty every time" — but "when the girls begin to smoke in public in this neighborhood the police will simply raid the place." He insisted he did not want women to think he was not their friend. In conclusion Big Tim told the reporter, "I hope women won't smoke in public. It's only that Little Tim and me were both born here and we love New York, and we want to keep it pure and as good as we can. Those things are all right for Paris, but New York ain't Paris — not by a long shot."[40]

Three years later, in the fall of 1911, New York City aldermen were reportedly intent of finding out if the rumors that women smoked in public places in the city were true, and if those stories were true to try to legislate an end to it. With that aim in mind, Alderman Dowling offered a resolution that directed the Corporation Counsel to advise the Board of

Aldermen as to its power to prohibit tobacco smoking by females in public places by legislative enactment. That resolution was adopted unanimously.[41]

One month later the New York City Corporation Counsel put an end to the Board of Aldermen's desires when he informed them they had no legal right to stop women smoking in public places. He also ruled that women could smoke at will on the city streets, be it cigarette, cigar, or pipe. At the same time, in Washington, D.C., E. H. Thomas, Corporation Counsel of the District of Columbia, stated that "no matter what blasé New Yorkers may do, Washingtonians of the gentler sex must not smoke while dining in public" when he ruled it acceptable for restaurants, and so on, to enact rules prohibiting women from smoking within their premises. Thomas allowed there could be no legal objection to women smoking in the streets of Washington, but he considered such an idea as "frivolous" and did not entertain it as a serious possibility of happening.[42]

In Kansas, Mrs. W. A. Johnston of Topeka—wife of Chief Justice Johnston—went before the Labor Legislative Committee of Kansas early in 1917 and obtained a promise of its cooperation to secure the passage of a law making cigarette advertising in newspapers and magazines a crime punishable by a fine and/or jail time. Under the proposal the law did not extend beyond cigarettes; left out were ads for pipe tobacco, chewing tobacco, cigars, and so forth.[43]

Although the opponents of cigarette smoking made some gains in this period, there were rollbacks of past gains as antipathy toward the cigarette eased, even in advance of the major rehabilitation in status wrought by World War I. In states that had banned possession of cigarettes, the courts often proved unwilling to apply the law to consumers, who were then free to obtain smokes by mail. Even dealers found that they were unlikely to be prosecuted, and cigarette consumption climbed despite the bans, even in the states where the sale of cigarettes was theoretically illegal. Indiana admitted defeat in 1909 and repealed its ban on cigarette sales, leaving a bar on sales to minors. Washington state followed in 1911, Minnesota in 1913, Wisconsin and Oklahoma in 1915, and South Dakota in 1917—all repealed bans on sales of cigarettes to adults. Getting such laws enacted, under pressure, was easy enough for groups that lobbied persistently, but getting those statutes enforced was a different matter. When World War I gave another boost to the popularity of cigarettes the opposition movement seemed to be on the ropes. But in 1919 the 18th Amendment to the Constitution (women's suffrage) was ratified by the states; that gave the anticigarette movement a boost, for it was widely believed that once women got the vote a great many problems would be solved.[44]

During this period, smoking by women had made great gains in the sense that it had come to be grudgingly accepted in public places, such as restaurants and the common areas of hotels, but still not on the street, or in other public places, such as railroads. The coming period, 1919–1927, would see a further expansion of female smoking into public spaces and a spread throughout various strata of society. In the 1920s, for example, a huge debate was under way on smoking in universities and colleges by female students. By and large women had their way. It was a significant step as cigarettes enticed the young females who were members of the intelligentsia — the future leaders and trendsetters of female society.

9

Abroad, 1919–1927

"To smoke in public is always bad taste in a woman. In private she may be pardoned if she does it with sufficient elegance."
— Alexandre Duval, 1921

A report from England in 1920 stated that women smoked practically everywhere since the war and that in the streets "Englishmen have become quite accustomed to having women ask them for a light." Supposedly the emancipated English woman had invaded men's territory to such an extent that on the golf links and in hotels it was at times possible to find posted notices that read, "This smoking room is reserved for gentlemen only."[1]

Later that same year customs officials at French ports were said to be refusing women the right accorded to male travelers of bringing a certain quantity of cigarettes for personal use into the country. It was done on the ground that French women were "not supposed to smoke."[2]

French women were increasingly turning to cigarettes at that time, which caused one commentator to remark that even middle-class French women, "among the most conservative and properly behaved in the world — seem to be fast succumbing to the smoking habit, in which English and American women have set the example." However, to that point their smoking was claimed to be a very private affair with the habit being practiced by them in the seclusion of their own homes. In restaurants and public places only American and English women were declared to smoke, "and those French women who do not belong to any social world. No well-bred French woman of the same class as those English and American women who thus transgress would think of doing so." As the prevalence of women smoking increased, protests were lodged by men with many of them having been shocked by the number of American and English women who in

94

the last season had indulged in cigarette smoking in public "with a freedom a Frenchman associates only with Bohemia and the demi-monde." Alexandre Duval, a well-known restaurateur and described as one of the last of the "dandies," asserted: "To smoke in public is always bad taste in a woman. In private she may be pardoned if she does it with sufficient elegance."[3]

By 1921 a comment was made that the woman who smoked while she shopped had been seen lately in the West End of London and that a well-known political hostess was often to be seen shopping while smoking a cigarette held in a long holder. One observer felt that practice would not be welcomed from the perspective of being a fire hazard and that objections would be raised from other women who did not like tobacco and would no more enter a shop that allowed smoking than they would enter a smoking carriage when traveling by train. According to this account, men accompanying women shopping in the West End generally, as a matter of courtesy, discarded their cigar or cigarette before going into "a strictly feminine domain, and their action may be held to express the point of view of the vast majority of women. The habit ought to be discouraged, as highly dangerous to property and offensive to the majority of shoppers."[4]

In a Dublin court in 1922, the question was raised as to whether females should be allowed to smoke at work during office hours. Miss Smith, a bookkeeper, was in court claiming a week's wages in lieu of notice from her employers who had fired her for smoking a cigarette during working hours. Smith said that all the male workers in the office smoked during work hours. Her claim to a week's pay was granted by the court.[5]

Men who habitually traveled in the smoking compartments on English trains were said to be demanding in 1923 that space be set aside and labeled "For Men Only" because women were usurping the smokers. Soon after women became enfranchised, a cry went up from those in favor of equal rights for compartments for the use of women only. Railways complied with that request but then the men complained because, they said, women walked right past empty and partly empty "Ladies Only" compartments and sat in the smoker compartments. Worse still, groaned the men, some of those women did not even smoke.[6]

During the Royal Ascot horse race in London in June 1924, a sensation of the day was the issuance of strict orders against women smoking in the royal enclosure. It had always been understood that women invited to the enclosure, which was just in front of the royal box, should not indulge in smoking while within range of the queen's eyes, and until this particular day that unwritten law had been obeyed. But among the 6,000 invitations issued to the enclosure for 1924, one was apparently sent to a woman who was not acquainted with the rules of behavior required there, or who was "daring." Royal court officials were described as "horrified" to witness a flagrant breach of etiquette on the part of a visitor not very far from the royal box when the unidentified woman lit up and smoked a cigarette, and on the following day those officials issued strict instructions to all the attendants to see the offense was not repeated.[7]

While opposition to female smoking was very muted abroad compared to that which existed in America, it was not absent. An antitobacco movement, the Union of Enemies of Tobacco, was launched in Leipzig, Germany, in summer 1924. Especially unsettling to the group was the issue of smoking among German women, which the group contended was spreading at an alarming rate. Estimates were that many thousands of German women aged 15 to 50 had taken to cigarettes within the previous few years. The group proposed, by law or otherwise, to make cigarette smoking less popular among the women and after that strategy had been successful, then to move on to the male smokers with the ultimate goal being to banish tobacco smoking altogether.[8]

Lady Astor had her say in London in 1925 in a budget debate in the House of Commons. Under debate was a proposal to remove certain taxation from tobacco and alcohol. She told Mr. Guinness, financial secretary of the Treasury, that she hoped he would not encourage smoking by lowering tobacco taxes, stating she was "horrified that the great and good Liberal Party should put forward a scheme to encourage smoking." Defending the idea was Liberal MP Hore Belissa, who commented that tobacco use was growing among women and the Chancellor of the Exchequer had already penalized women by taxing their silk stockings and lace "and in continuing tobacco duty he is making life well-nigh impossible for them."[9]

When America's Bryn Mawr College for women changed its smoking rules in 1925, the story was featured in the English newspapers but not on the basis that allowing female students to smoke was a radical idea, because women's colleges and schools in the United Kingdom were said to have permitted smoking for years. At the University of London, several thousand women had their own little clubs where they could puff away at will while not in class. The London County Council, which conducted night classes attended by 26,000 women, permitted them to smoke in various areas, but not in class. Smoking was not encouraged among public school girls nor among those in private colleges where the students were in their teens, said the report, but there was no ban in any of the educational institutions for students aged 20 and over.[10]

Around 1926 women smokers were said to be invading previously exclusively male London smoking cafés. Said the director of a firm that operated 50 smoking cafés in the London city district, "A few years ago no woman would ever have dared pass our doors. Today we could not keep them out if we tried!" He added that a few years earlier if a woman smoker did succeed in entering, "we certainly would not have permitted her to indulge in a cigarette — not even a scented one with a strip of pink satin around the end." Unhappily, he reported, everything was then different. "Women have been smoking for years — at homes, at

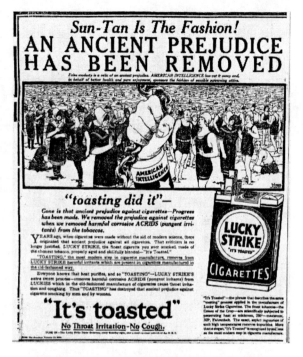

The bottom line in this 1926 ad declared the ancient preudice against smoking cigarettes by men and women had been destroyed.

dances and in the cafés and restaurants of the West End, but lately they have even swarmed into the smoking cafés of the city which, even after smoking for women had received universal sanction, were by common consent regarded as the exclusive resort of men." Also, it was said that many businesswomen and female office workers in London were adopting the 11 o'clock coffee and cigarette habit, and some employers allowed them a 10-minute interval for that specific purpose.[11]

When the London-based British American Tobacco Company announced its profits for 1926 were over six million pounds sterling, one million pounds more than in 1925, it attributed those increased profits to the growth of the smoking habit among women.[12]

10

America, 1919–1927

> *"The college is certain that there is not a School Board in Michigan that would elect as teacher a young woman who smoked cigarettes if it knew she did so."*
> — Charles McKenny, Michigan State
> Normal School President, 1922

> *"It may be true that women have the same rights as men to drink and smoke and indulge habits peculiar to masculinity, but that means the lowering of the standards of womanhood to the level of the men."*
> — Buffalo, New York, *Evening Post*, 1925

No aspect of the issue of women smoking received as much attention in the United States in the 1920s as did the question of smoking in the colleges and universities and whether the female students should smoke — at both the women-only colleges and at coed institutions. It all started quietly enough in late February 1919, when the students at Vassar College in Poughkeepsie, New York, went on record as being opposed to women smoking, following a meeting of the students at the women-only facility. After discussing the question, they voted their disapproval of the practice of women smoking. Burgess Johnson, a professor in the English department and director of publicity at the college explained, "They voted against the proposition; I am told. I have not heard of any of the students smoking and the students have never asked permission to smoke."[1]

Eighteen months later P. V. Hocking authored an article vehemently opposed to the practice in Stanford University's *Pictorial* publication. First, he noted many women were smoking at Stanford, with an especially big increase among those females newly arrived. If women wanted to smoke he felt they should do it in private; "If women are accustomed to smoking in their own homes or around the San Francisco hotels, that is their own business, but to quote an old adage — When in Rome do as the Romans do." Hocking argued further that Stanford had neither the right nor the desire to meddle with anyone's habits outside of the university, "but when women come here they are expected to maintain the standards of conduct laid down by the university, which standards are made by people whose judgment is far superior to theirs and are merely those statements of good form which no woman who considers herself a lady can possibly violate." As far as he was concerned if any woman at the California facility did not care to accept those standards of conduct then they should leave, "and the quicker the better." Vassar was cited by Hocking as a college that had faced the issue and successfully settled it, claiming the practice there had been all but eradicated. "Stanford will do the same," he fulminated. Without giving any details he said several women had already left Stanford, "by request," for smoking. Hocking warned women students, "Stanford University is no place to bring the accursed weed.... In closing the women should be reminded that they will immediately be expelled if caught smoking and this verdict will be upheld by the women of this university. You just can't do it.... It doesn't get by."[2]

University of Chicago president Harry Pratt Judson banned smoking in women's dormitories in December 1921. Accustomed to making their own rules, the dormitory women suddenly were confronted with a notice from the house mothers against the cigarette. No explanation was officially offered, but rumor had it that the dean of women and others on the campus had protested against what was considered excessive smoking by women students.[3]

As 1922 began the debate intensified. A reporter doing a round-up article on the topic began his piece by saying that smoking by females was "a vile, dirty and vulgar habit" that should be prohibited in every university but was hard to regulate, according to the deans of women at the University of Chicago and Northwestern University. Marion Talbot, dean of women at the University of Chicago, said the institution had no regulations against smoking by coeds because "although it is a filthy habit, it is almost impossible to prevent it and there is little use in trying." (The ban by Judson was not mentioned and presumably it had fallen by the wayside.) Dean Mary Ross at Northwestern said she had issued stringent rules against smoking by coeds. Although there was no rule prohibiting smoking by women at the University of Wisconsin (Madison), F. Louise Nardin, dean of women, stated there was an ethical principle held by coeds that was making the habit unpopular. Nardin felt that smoking females belonged to the "idle, blasé disappointed class." An intelligent woman, she declared, "cannot see herself rocking a baby or making a pie with a cigarette in her mouth, flicking ashes in the baby's face or dropping them in the pie crust." In closing she argued, "I do not think the habit is regarded as smart at Wisconsin any longer. It rather has come to be regarded as vulgar." Mrs. Jessie Ladd, dean of women at the University of Minnesota (Minneapolis), believed smoking by coeds at universities was practiced just to be "smart" and that there was very little of it at her university. Although there was no rule forbidding the practice, the sororities at Minnesota had all spoken against it, remarked Ladd.[4]

Continuing on with the survey, Anne Blitz, dean of women at the University of Kansas, explained there was no rule against smoking by women students there because such a rule was unnecessary. "Smoking by women here is a negligible problem. The sororities here have strict rules against smoking and enforce them." About one percent of coeds at Ohio University (Columbus) smoked, according to Louise Brown, acting dean of women. Every effort was made by the women's department, she said, to discourage smoking among female students. "It is a dirty habit," said Brown, "harmful not only to girls who smoke but in the effects on those who see them." Also, householders who lodged coeds were urged to ban smoking, Brown commented, and when it became known a female smoked she was called before the dean and efforts were made to show her why she should not. According to the view of Elizabeth Hoskins, dean of women at the University of Louisville, smoking by university coeds was simply a fad that would soon pass. "I can't feel that a real, genuine womanly girl would form the habit," she said. There had been no cases of smoking among women students at the university, said Hoskins, because the South is a "little more conservative than the North." A coed caught smoking at Purdue University (Lafayette, Indiana) would be dismissed from the university at once, said Caroline Shoemaker, dean of women there. However, she added, no case of a female student smoking had been reported. J. S. Gau, spokesperson for the University of Pittsburgh, explained that a no-smoking rule existed for coeds, but "if smoking by girls is going on, it is so small as hardly worthy of attention."[5]

Around the same time a different account reported little student smoking at California institutes of higher learning. Smoking had not become a habit, or even a condoned fad, among women students of Western universities was the emphatic assertion of Olive Presler, president of the Associated Women Students of the University of California. Commenting because of news dispatches about the existence of the habit in Midwestern universities, Presler stated she knew personally more than half of the 5,000 female students in the University of California system and of that number she knew not even one who had ever smoked. Smoking, she explained, was not allowed in the sorority houses or women's clubs and the coeds' code of honor forbade the practice. At the last conference of the Western Intercollegiate Association of Women Students, in Berkeley, Presler said a frank discussion of smoking was held, "and it was agreed that there was nothing to be feared from smoking among college women in the West."[6]

Instructors at any of the state normal colleges in Nebraska were informed in February 1922 that hereafter they would be refused leaves of absence to study or attend Columbia University, the University of Chicago, or Northwestern University "because of testimony of those who have been students and the news items in the daily press show that cigarette smoking is common among women in these institutions," according to a press account. That action was then taken in a resolution adopted by the board of education of the state normal schools. Columbia University (New York) officials characterized the action as "regrettable." Charles T. MacFarlane, Columbia controller of teachers' colleges, issued a public statement repudiating an announcement made a few days earlier by Margaret Kilpatrick, president of the Whittier Hall (Columbia) student body to the effect that smoking in the women's rooms was prohibited, but only because the smoke made the rooms too stuffy. Worried that statement by Kilpatrick was one of the news items that led to the Nebraska action, MacFarlane insisted, "Smoking by women in Whittier Hall is forbidden for moral, not architectural reasons."[7]

Not all female residences at Columbia barred smoking, though. Students living at Brooks Hall, a women's dormitory, had settled the question for themselves. As one of them explained, "The matter was left for the student body to decide and we voted unanimously to allow smoking in the bedrooms, in the parlors and in the banquet halls." Fernald Hall, which was the dorm where graduate students lived, along with others taking extension course at Columbia, had no rules against smoking. One student who lived there said females smoked in their rooms and that some of them smoked in Columbia Commons, one of the large dining halls where they went for meals; Fernald Hall had no dining rooms. At a banquet given by Barnard alumnae, cigarettes were passed with the coffee and, according to one of the guests, "only a few refused them." That caused a journalist to comment that such behavior seemed to indicate that the arbitrary ruling of college faculties in the past against smoking had not succeeded in eradicating a taste for cigarettes.[8]

Wellesley College was another female institution that followed the idea of student self-government in certain areas. Students who disobeyed the Undergraduate Association's regulation against smoking were requested to leave the college. The matter was handled entirely through the student body, and it was said that few members defied the ruling against smoking. Abuses of former years when the women smoked behind locked, cotton-padded doors, were declared to be fast disappearing. At Vassar, where the female student body had also voted down smoking on campus and in the dormitories, the offense was punished with expulsion, "But the Faculty has nothing whatever to do with the question, which is settled entirely by the student body." Supposedly smoking among the students had ceased without the friction that existed in the old days, when boards comprised of teachers sat in judgment on students who had allegedly violated rules. Bryn Mawr was another Eastern college that expelled students for ciga-rette smoking, but left the matter to the discretion of the self-governing committee. Said a matron of one of the dorms at the all-women institute, "the charm of cigarette smoking, like other mooted questions, will only be enhanced by college legislation against it. The students are quite able to decide the question for themselves and the only regulations of any value are those passed by the governing student body."[9]

An announcement was made in April 1922 by Charles McKenny, pres-ident, and Bessie Leach Priddy, dean of women, that 17 women students at Michigan State Normal College (Ypsilanti) had been expelled, many because of smoking. Some of the females were asked to leave school because "indignant" landladies caught them smoking cigarettes in the pri-vate houses where they lodged. (Others were expelled for other indiscre-tions, such as climbing through a window after the front door had been locked.) Members of the faculty reportedly supported McKenny and Priddy in the disciplinary action, arguing the misdemeanors were harmful because they resulted in poor classwork. Also, many of the faculty made it plain, said a reporter, that they believed bobbed hair, cigarettes, and strolling in gardens under the moon "did not fall short of being actually sinful, intol-erable on their own account and certainly unbecoming to a woman." McKenny's statement on the disciplinary action declared the position of the college was that the people of the state of Michigan supported the Michigan State Normal College for the training of teachers and they had a right to say what kind of teachers they wanted in their schools. "The col-lege is certain that there is not a School Board in Michigan that would elect as teacher a young woman who smoked cigarettes if it knew she did so," continued McKenny. "That being the case, the college will not knowingly permit any young woman to remain in school, much less graduate here, who smokes tobacco, and moreover it will consider no house a proper place for its young women to room that permits girls to smoke. Until the people of Michigan change their attitude and are willing to take women smokers as teachers the college will adhere to this policy."[10]

Alice Tanton was one of the students expelled by McKenny for allegedly smoking cigarettes. She sued the college to compel them to readmit her in a case that attracted statewide attention. Tanton contended cigarette butts found in her room in the wastebasket had been used to char the edges of posters on the walls of her room — that is, she did not smoke those cigarettes but only used them in an artistic manner. Also, Tanton contended there was no specific rule against cigarette smoking at the school and that the authorities were discriminating in seeking to make a requirement for females that they did not make for males. Two years after expulsion, in March 1924, Tanton's dismissal from college was upheld by the Michigan State Supreme Court in a decision handed down in Lansing. At the time Tanton was working as a stenographer in Detroit. Not only did the Supreme Court refuse to grant a readmission order, it praised college officials for "maintaining certain ideals" for the young women who would become the teachers of the state and declared that instead of condemning dean of women Priddy, "she should be commended for upholding some of the old-fashioned ideals of young womanhood." Priddy was then employed at the University of Missouri and just a few days before the Tanton decision she again came before the public eye when she caused the expulsion of 11 students (4 of them females) from that institution on charges of drinking liquor.[11]

Writing in the *Ladies Home Journal* in 1922, journalist Harry Burke told the story of Mr. and Mrs. John Smith from the Midwest who were visiting New York City mainly to see their daughter, then attending a Manhattan college. Mr. Smith was described as a life-long smoker while Mrs. Smith was a nonsmoker and, at home, an active member of the YWCA and the Anti-Cigarette League. For her the sight of women smoking cigarettes, said Burke, "was so repellent that she refused to enter any of the dining rooms of the hotel. The Smiths had their meals served in their rooms." They were horrified to learn their daughter Eleanor had taken up smoking. Then they learned that in her school there was a room set aside for smoking; the school did not allow smoking in class or in the dorm rooms. Visiting the school the next day, a spokesman explained to the Smiths, regarding the female students, that they came from the best families in America with some of them permitted by their parents to smoke in their own homes. "It is a modern idea we do not approve of, and we were reluctant to make any concession here, but for the sake of discipline it had to be done," explained the spokesman. "We found that in spite of all our precautions some of the girls smoked in their rooms. So we set aside a room and told the young women that if they wanted to smoke they could do so in that room. We put them on their honor to smoke there and there only." He felt that way the college was able to watch them and to prevent any excesses as well as the "contamination" of the nonsmokers.[12]

On November 8, 1922, Vassar students voted to continue their self-imposed rule against smoking. An amendment was suggested that would have allowed juniors and seniors to smoke and permitted the practice at certain parties. However, that amendment was also voted down.[13]

Things quieted down for a brief period as the topic received minimal attention, until it erupted anew as a hot topic in 1925. Early that year West Virginia University (Morgantown) president Dr. F. B. Trotter stated the school was taking disciplinary action against women students who smoked, although he declined to say whether any students had been expelled for that offense. One female was disciplined by being denied permission to attend a military ball at the school because she had smoked, but was allowed to stay in school on the condition that she promise not to smoke again. "We have always had a rule against smoking by women students," said Trotter, "and when violators are brought before me I try to make the discipline conform to the character of the case and the circumstances surrounding it."[14]

Vassar continued to bar smoking. Under a resolution passed by the Students' Assembly in February 1925 and ratified by the Student Council, smoking remained forbidden in any Vassar College building. The resolution declared that since smoking was not yet established as a social convention acceptable to all groups throughout the country, it was therefore not approved at Vassar. Underlying the resolution, said officers of the Students' Association, was the fact that letters from every part of the country had shown that smoking by women was not yet sufficiently approved to be accepted by Vassar without "seriously menacing the best interests of the college."[15]

All college precedents in New England were said to have been broken in October 1925, when the Massachusetts Institute of Technology (MIT) announced that henceforth females would be permitted to smoke at dances and other social events in the Walker Memorial Building, where undergraduate social events were held. There were only a few women students at MIT, but the rule applied to them as well as to female guests of the male students at dances. The question of women smoking had been debated for months and had caused much dissension. Finally, the Institute Committee, which was the student governing council, determined there would be no ban against the use of cigarettes by women, in the context described. Meanwhile, smoking anywhere at any time was still forbidden to Wellesley and Radcliffe students and to females at Boston University. A violation of the rule at the latter school meant expulsion. Also at that time, the 800 women students at Goucher College (Baltimore, Maryland) were busy studying their school's 1925-1926 *Blue Book of Social Regulations.* Under those rules, upper-class members could go riding with a gentleman, but not after six p.m., and then only if he was approved and if she promised not to stray beyond the bounds of Baltimore or its suburbs. Contained within the regulations was a list of the seven approved restaurants and tea-rooms in Baltimore to which students could go without seeking permission. Two theaters and six cinemas were also on the approved list. Smoking was covered by this rule: "No student shall smoke in the college buildings or in public places in the city of Baltimore."[16]

Changes in the no-smoking rules continued to occur. Around March 1925, Vassar College announced that its official position was one of disapproval of smoking as injurious to health but left it with the conscience of students to determine whether or not they would continue the self-imposed prohibition. In response to a questionnaire, 433 students said they smoked (45 percent) and 524 said they did not. Yet they voted "overwhelmingly" in favor of modifying the blanket ban against smoking. Henceforth smoking by students at Vassar would be permitted in certain specific sections of the campus—but not in dorm rooms or in dining rooms.[17]

In the fall of 1925, female students from Wellesley, Radcliffe, Jackson College, Simmons College, and Boston University were forbidden by their administration officials to attend the upcoming Harvard-Yale dance, as well as all such social events in the future, including the Harvard-Dartmouth dance. Official explanations as to the reasons for the action were vague, mentioning that the dances had nothing to do with the colleges in question and "they are of an extremely questionable nature owing to the fact that they are entirely open to the public." Any student who disobeyed would be disciplined, although it was said such punishment would not be so severe as to include expulsion. A rumor as to the real reason for the ban related, "It is said that hints of cigarette smoking and partaking from flasks had come to the attention of the college officials."[18]

A proposal to permit smoking by Wellesley College students when off the campus was defeated by the Senate of the College Government Association. The five faculty members of the Senate voted down the proposal, against the affirmative votes of the three student delegates. Some time earlier that resolution had been passed by the other branch of the student government body and had been endorsed by 82 percent of the 1,207 students who voted in a referendum on the subject. That action by the Senate left in place the old, existing rule that forbade students to smoke anywhere "while living under the regulations of the College Government

Association." In a public statement explaining their vote the five faculty members said, "True progress demands that a college community should not follow doubtful social conventions but should exert its influence to maintain high standards of living.... To sanction smoking is contrary to the spirit and traditions of the college, which are a valued possession of more than the present college generation."[19]

Still in 1925, it became known that students at Mount Holyoke and Smith Colleges favored a modification of the college restriction on smoking. In a referendum the Mount Holyoke women voted 448 to 442 on a proposal to revise the existing rule, which forbade smoking while under the college jurisdiction. Only 27 voted for the right to smoke anywhere any time, and 327 favored the Vassar system, permitting smoking in some specified section of the college grounds. Women at Smith had decided to let the issue rest until a new honor system agreement was drawn up in the following spring, when, it was reported, there would be an attempt to establish a rule similar to the one at Vassar. As the matter stood Smith women were pledged not to smoke anywhere on campus or in the community of Northampton (Massachusetts), wherein Smith was located.[20]

Barnard College (all female) had never questioned the right of young women to smoke, according to a statement from Miss M. V. Libby, assistant to the dean. Officially, Barnard had never opposed the practice. Smoking was not permitted in the Administration Building, but that was largely a fire prevention measure, said Libby. It was left to the students themselves to say whether smoking would be allowed elsewhere. Students were permitted to smoke in the dormitory rooms. Also, they voted as to whether they would smoke in the study rooms. Libby said that some years they voted yes on the matter and some years they voted no. As the study rooms were used by many students at the same time, it was left to the student body to regulate their use. Although Barnard had never had any rule against the practice, on the other hand, the habit was discouraged by medical lecturers there as injurious to health. Smoking remained prohibited at Radcliffe with a reported agitation for the lifting of that ban being unsuccessful in spring 1925.[21]

One of the most significant and well-publicized events of the time came in Bryn Mawr, Pennsylvania, in November 1925. The Self-Government Association of all-female Bryn Mawr College (an organization containing all undergraduates as members and solely responsible for the conduct of students) had found it increasingly impossible to enforce the rule against smoking. Therefore the association petitioned college president Marion Edwards Park to permit smoking, under certain restrictions. Under an order issued by Park on November 23, one room was set aside as a smoking-permitted area in each hall of residence, and also allowed on the lower athletic field when games were not in progress. In changing the rule, Park issued a statement explaining the conduct of the Bryn Mawr students had always been in the hands of the association and their regulations had been based on public opinion of the time. "Such public opinion in a college democracy is controlled in larger matters by conscience and in lesser matters by convention. As early as 1897 the regulation against smoking was made and has been in effect up to this time," Park continued. "A change in the attitude toward smoking by women has come in twenty-five years and is naturally reflected among college students. A regulation prohibiting smoking can no longer depend on the authority of conscience and convention, which makes up public opinion, and it is no longer effective." Another reason, she explained, was that as attempts to enforce the no-smoking rule increasingly failed it began to affect student relations to other regulations and that the old rule stood apart from other regulations in the sense that "it is no longer resting solidly on intelligent public opinion." A questionnaire sent out to students revealed that many supporters of the change were not themselves smokers, and that less than half of the student body smoked.[22]

Following the Bryn Mawr decision, Mr. A. T. Allen, superintendent of public instruction in Raleigh, North Carolina, said he felt Bryn Mawr had taken the lead and other women's colleges would soon follow that example. "I see no reason why women should not smoke as well as men," he said. "It is merely a part of the general breaking down of differences between the sexes."[23]

An editorial in the *Washington Post* on the Bryn Mawr decision felt that no matter how much it was to be regretted that college women smoked, it was better they should indulge openly than to do it on the sly, away from the eyes of the officials. "It is not impossible that the removal of the prohibition will cause the young women the sooner to grow tired of the habit, which is not natural to the sex," hoped the editor.[24]

Bryn Mawr's move sparked much media attention, drawing a wide range of reaction. The Utica, New York, *Press* offered the thought that colleges were presumed to promote intellectual honesty and Bryn Mawr had shown it was honest, at the least, while the Philadelphia *Bulletin* declared Park's reasoning was sound because the experience of every college head was that an unenforceable regulation led to the formation of secret practices and tended to weaken other discipline. Pittsburgh's *Gazette Times* agreed it was better the students smoke openly than secretly. However, Mary Towle, a Bryn Mawr grad and then assistant district attorney, expressed regret because she disliked women smoking in public and "instinctively" regretted it had received the endorsement of a college like her alma mater. She thought smoking "is purely a question of taste, with no moral or ethical elements involved." Also unhappy was the Indianapolis *Star*, which said its part of the country still looked askance at the woman who indulged in public. Grudgingly, it added, "Young girls think it smart; some women think it Bohemian. Others enjoy smoking and see no reason why they should be criticized. Their argument does not readily admit an answer." Most people regarded the issue not so much as one of right or wrong but as one of good taste or bad taste, declared the Pittsburgh *Post*. It was a moral question only as it might affect the health. Yet it was hardly conceivable to the *Post* that anyone would desire a woman or girl in whose welfare he was interested to take up smoking. "A passive attitude, an acquiescent attitude, may be taken in regard to it; but no father or mother, no husband, no brother would deliberately set about to persuade a woman member of his family to smoke as he might set about to persuade her to dance or to play cards. There is a world of significance in that." Harshest of all was the Buffalo, *Evening Post*, which argued, "The coarsening effect upon young womanhood through the smoking of cigarettes, through the exposure of nakedness in public appearance, of over painting the face and lips, and of petting parties, are everywhere apparent." This editor added, "It may be true that women have the same rights as men to drink and smoke and indulge habits peculiar to masculinity, but that means the lowering of the standards of womanhood to the level of the men."[25]

Under the old Bryn Mawr rule, students were not allowed to smoke within 25 miles of the college, except in private homes where smoking was thought proper and allowed by the householder. Any girl breaking the rule was bound in honor to report her misdemeanor to the Executive Board, which meted out such punishment as it saw fit. Reportedly, culprits turned themselves in, "as a matter of course." That is, they did until around the start of 1925, when the arrangement began to break down significantly; "Though culprits were numerous, penitents were few," wrote an observer. Though the women were said to be as honorable as ever, they had simply formed a new notion of what constituted their bound duty. Student leaders talked it over and decided that when a law ceased to be respected, something was wrong with the law. A questionnaire was sent out to 386 undergraduates asking if they favored the existing regulation or wanted a new rule. Although less than half smoked, 321 favored a new rule, only 46 opposed it — the new rule was to allow smoking in certain common rooms but not in the dorm rooms. A *New York Times* reporter, puzzled as to why women wanted to smoke, offered the following: "By some queer alchemy the cigarette has become her symbol of freedom. It isn't the cigarette that she wants. It is rather what the cigarette represents. And she is essentially honest. Since it isn't honest to smoke when smoking is against the rule, she would alter the rule." He believed that college women who wanted to smoke for the sake of smoking were very few in number. When the Bryn Mawr news broke, students at Smith College circulated petitions to change their rules. But in the previous year the Student Government Association had put in place a much-revised code of regulations and it wanted to give that code at least a full year trial. One rule read, "Members of the student body are not allowed to smoke except on out-of-town blue card privileges." That meant they could not smoke in the community of Northampton, but when at home or visiting in places approved by their parents they were free to act as they and their parents saw fit.[26]

Cigarette smoking was not permitted or tolerated among women or men students in the buildings or on the campus of the Central State Normal School at Edmond, Oklahoma, and students were given to understand that it was against the rules of student boardinghouses. Of course, a teacher training facility in 1920s America contained no male students, or very close to it. According to college president John G. Mitchell, only twice in five years had the rule been violated. On average, fall, winter and spring attendance of young women at Central was 800, with the average summer attendance being 1,700 women. No numbers were given for males. Not only were students given to understand that cigarette smoking would "under no circumstances be tolerated," said Mitchell, "but they are taught that it is immodest and detrimental to health."[27]

In a 1925 survey of parents of college women on the question of whether those women should smoke, the fathers and mothers of students at the Boston University College of Practical Arts and Letters registered an emphatic *no*. A questionnaire was sent to 675 parents of the students in that department of the university by Dean T. Lawrence Davis. Returned surveys numbered 450 and only one of them failed to take a definite stand against females smoking. Several of the letters said the writers positively would not permit their daughters to attend an institution where smoking was permitted. "My feeling in the matter is that girls of college age should not be permitted to decide this matter for themselves," Davis said. "Our rule against smoking will continue to be rigidly enforced, and the penalty for infraction is expulsion. For most of the girls the rule is no hardship; they have no desire to smoke." A sample from the comments written on the questionnaires by the parents included, "Smoking removes the sweetness and charm which goes with girls' femininity," "It is well to remember that the girls in your college from 1925 to 1929 will be the mothers of the girls in your college in 1950; and I am sure that cigarette smoking does not lead to the highest type of motherhood," "I feel that a girl who smokes is lowering her resistance to the temptations which constantly surround her. What she learns by submitting to discipline will in later years become a pleasant habit," "I have never been able to dissociate female cigarette smokers from people of the red light strata of society," "We heartily endorse your attitude. A great deal of this talk about personal freedom is propaganda badly tainted with Bolshevism. The immature mind cannot readily penetrate the mazes of sophistry. As a matter of fact, we have no personal freedom in the strict sense. Society is much safer for these restrictions," "We surely are living in peculiar times when the Christian dean of a Christian college should have to ask the support of parents regarding the fearful evil that the so-called smart young women are taking up in our institutions of learning," "I admire the stand which you are taking in this matter. Parents who have a grain of common sense are getting tired of paying out money for giving children college educations and having them turned out flappers and cigarette fiends. The money comes hard and the colleges ought to feel bound to teach the right kind of things," "Smoking on the part of an intelligent girl indicates weak character. Smoking because of fear of being socially disapproved is an act of cowardice and shows lack of independence," and

> As you know, there are physiological reasons why young women, the mothers of future America, should not smoke. To these, of course, one must add the moral and esthetic. The average young man thinks he can take greater liberties with the girl who smokes. To that extent the effect is demoralizing and tends to deprive the gentler sex of that refining, edifying influence which now, more than ever, is essential to the welfare of America's young manhood.[28]

The clubhouse of the woman's faculty at the University of California at Berkeley decided early in 1926 to permit smoking and to offer cigarettes for sale. Explaining the move was Marian Ransome, manager of the clubhouse, who said the impetus was "irresistible demand." She added, "It was the only thing we could do. Members of the club are mature women and certainly know whether they want to smoke."[29]

The Students' Association at Vassar College voted in 1926 to set aside a conference room in the student building where undergrads could smoke, free from the restrictions that had been placed on the practice on the immediate campus. The senior students also received permission to smoke in the senior parlor in Main Hall. The action of the association in permitting smoking under those conditions was considered a revolutionary step. For a year, a courtesy rule had been in force prohibiting smoking in the buildings and "frowning severely" on smoking openly on the campus. Vassar seemed to have tried to appear liberal by not prohibiting the practice in certain sections of the campus (apparently all outdoors), but at the same time it tried to load so much guilt and psychological pressure on any woman who dared try that it would have a de facto prohibition.[30]

With respect to Bryn Mawr and Vassar having set examples by allowing their students to smoke, with some restrictions, a *New York Times* editor worried the use of tobacco would become a habit in college precincts generally. On the Vassar move in particular the editor declared, "The new rule is a surrender of the college authorities in spite of the President's disclaimer of responsibility" (arguing students governed themselves). Smoking by Vassar students was still forbidden in the dorm rooms, on the immediate campus, or in restaurants in Poughkeepsie and in neighboring towns. Warned the editor, "It is one of the most improbable things in the world that the women will surrender their right to smoke."[31]

Dr. Rufus B. Von Kleinsmid banned smoking in 1926 at the University of Southern California (Los Angeles). In the opinion of A. G. Paul, dean of the Riverside Junior College, such an edict would mean nothing in Riverside, California, because smoking "simply wasn't done by female students at the Riverside School.... At that, I believe the percentage of girl smokers at California colleges is small."[32]

Cigarettes in the mouths of two student nurses at the Henry Ford Hospital School in Detroit resulted in such an upheaval that Mr. W. L. Graham, the superintendent of the school, and Katherine G. Kimmick, superintendent of nurses, "the highest paid nurse in the world," were no longer employed there. Miss Scarth and Miss Patterson, nurses of the senior class, were discovered smoking cigarettes in the nurses' residence in violation of a Ford rule. They were spotted by a Miss Bennett, an instructor, who reported the violation to Kimmick. When she called all the nurses together, she asked them what discipline should be applied to the two offenders. Reportedly the student body voted for severe discipline; Kimmick then expelled them. When the two punished students protested, Kimmick declared they would stay expelled or she would resign. Although the school gave no official reason as to why Kimmick was no longer employed there, rumor had it that the stand she took over the two nurses was the cause of her dismissal. Because the school's board would not discuss the matter at all, it was unknown whether Graham's dismissal was due to the smoking incident or not.[33]

President H. N. MacCracken of Vassar College stated in 1927 that a recent news dispatch from Louisville, Kentucky, had grossly misrepresented his attitude on the subject of women smoking. He indicated in fact that he would not dignify what he considered a social question of relatively little importance by assuming a public attitude toward it. MacCracken explained that he resented it when reporters sought to interview him regarding smoking at Vassar following his address before the Kentucky Educational Association. He added, "I requested not to be interviewed on the subject of women smoking and objected to the triviality of the question that was brought up at an important meeting of an educational character. I also unequivocally deny that I made the statement that the women should help the men to consume the tobacco crop of the country." What he had said was that as he understood it there was more objection to women smoking in those parts of the United States where tobacco was raised than in either the extreme East or extreme West of the United States. Apparently, a reporter added a remark of his own but attributed it to Mac-Cracken. That was, "Tobacco is one of the country's most important crops. The men can't smoke it all up. Why shouldn't the women help?" And then the whole issue faded away. But by then smoking by female students was commonly allowed in many schools, and often practiced at banning schools when the blind eye was turned.[34]

Within American society in general, the habit spread among women and the consumption of cigarettes in total by Americans grew dramatically. T. L. Hughes, chief of the tobacco section of the U.S. Commerce Department, cited in 1925 an increase in the number of women smokers as one of the likely explanations of the great increase in cigarette consumption in America. In the course of his duties he found 15 billion cigarettes were consumed in 1913; 63 billion in 1924, more than a fourfold gain. Large gains were noted in other countries as well, especially Japan where consumption moved from 7 billion to 23 billion over those same years. That Japanese rate of increase came close to matching the rate of increase in the United States, the world leader in that department.[35]

Yet in a retrospective study conducted in 1985, only about 5 percent of women who were in their 20s in 1925 admitted having smoked then. However, it was a study with a small number of subjects and, of course, subject to the frailties of the human memory. No reliable statistics existed, through to 1927, as to the number of women who were smokers. Even estimates were rarely offered. Much of the practice of the habit remained covert, making estimation even more difficult. The sole estimate that may have had some validity was the Bryn Mawr survey, which revealed about 45 percent of its student body smoked, although the definition they used for a person to be classified as a smoker was not given. Surprisingly, the increase in women smokers took place in the absence of any cigarette advertising targeted directly at women. Social scientist Michael Schudson examined two urban newspapers and a general circulation magazine and found no advertisements picturing women smoking before 1926.[36]

One area where smoking women showed up more frequently and in a changing context — an area related to advertising — was in the movies. In a resolution adopted February 28, 1922, in Chicago by the Board of Managers of the international Anti-Cigarette League was a plea for the elimination of cigarette smoking by women in the movies except "as the accompaniment of discreditable character." That resolution was forwarded to U.S. postmaster general Will Hays, who was to enter the motion picture industry a few days later, on March 4, to become its czar and to clean up a variety of matters that had left the industry open to much public criticism. He reigned for several decades. Hays was urged by the league to use his efforts in his new position of "immense influence" in the motion picture industry "to secure early and universal action in

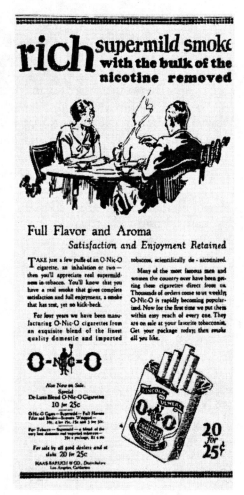

A woman as background in a 1927 ad.

accordance with this suggestion." According to the resolution, the appearance of cigarette-smoking women characters in films was described "of late as a growing habit among women of recognized respectability and among high school and college girls that threatens the element of womanhood that must mother the Americans of tomorrow."[37]

Another who was angry at the movies was Ernest Crutcher, a Los Angeles physician. He said the movies were hated by many who opposed cigarettes, not simply because the actresses used them, "but because of the suggestions conveyed to youthful audiences; the studied intent to impress upon them the chic, becoming, stylish, blasé, airy independence a cigarette carries to the simpleton who smokes one." Crutcher was incensed because "women are the precious caskets that bear through the ages the treasures of race heredity. They are the mothers of the race. Fancy a mother nursing a baby and smoking a filthy cigarette." He added, "It is not the maternal woman that smokes. It is the degraded types. A pure woman, if such takes up smoking, will soon take up other vices. Invariably! ... Tobacco evokes a moral debasement that is inescapable." Worst of all, warned Crutcher, "Roués know this; and where lust impels they have no hesitation to approach a female that smokes cigarettes. Tobacco stimulates the sexual passions while provoking a debility of powers."[38]

According to author Cassandra Tate, as cigarettes became more popular, the number of smokers in films increased, and their social status improved. Cigarettes were said to be rare in American films until the early 1920s, and usually signified vamping, or villainy. Sensitive to the imagery, the Tobacco Merchants Association protested in 1922 that only "the villain and every low type of character in the cast" smoked cigarettes, and that suggested to them that the habit was "confined to that class, hence is debasing. This is wrong, absolutely: it is unjust." The beginnings of the association between cigarette smoking and evil, wicked women in films went back to Theda Bara in *Carmen* (1915) and in *The Vixen* (1917). J. Stuart Blacton, a pioneering movie director, filmed a young man newly arrived in the sinful city (*On the Banks of the Wa-*

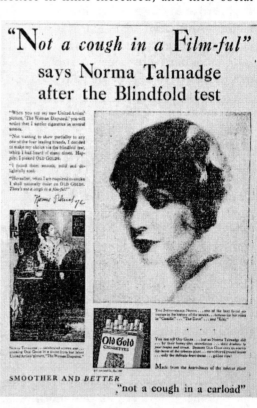

In this 1928 endorsement ad, actress Norma Talmadge got in a plug for her latest movie. This inset photograph was a still from that film while the text informed the reader that Talmadge smoked cigarettes in several scenes in that film, United Artists release *The Woman Disputed*.

bash, 1923) entering an apartment. The camera panned the back of the sofa as smoke curled upward from the opposite side. Then the viewers saw the head of a glamorous vamp rising to meet her visitor and, of course, to seduce, or vamp, him. On the basis of a scene in *Flesh and the Devil* (1926) in which she took a cigarette from the mouth of John Gilbert and struck a sexual pose, Greta Garbo was launched on the road to stardom. Among male characters in the movies a cigarette often gave visual evidence of degeneracy. In the silent film version of *Beau Geste* (1927) the evil character Lejaune smoked, not the noble Beau Geste. When Paramount remade *Beau Geste* with Gary Cooper in the title role in 1939, it was he who smoked while the evil Markov (the American version of Lejaune) did not smoke at all. That trend to having heroines and heroes smoke in films instead of the bad characters was foreshadowed in *A Woman of the World* (1926) wherein Pola Negri portrayed a worldly countess who visited relatives in a small Midwestern town. She arrived in the town, smoking a cigarette in a long holder, just as an antivice district attorney finished delivering a lecture on the evils of smoking. Eventually the Negri character humanized him and married him. At film's end he had given up his provincialism and intolerance while she continued smoking.[39]

Commenting on the increase in the number of women who smoked, a reporter visited tobacco shops in New York City in 1920 to determine how many women customers they had. At one shop he asked how many female customers they had in a day, wondering if it might be as high as 12 or 20. "Twelve or twenty? Seventy-five or a hundred is more like it," snapped the clerk. "They come in just the way men do. And they buy the same kind of cigarettes the men do." Referring again to the reporter's suggested numbers, the clerk added, "We had that number even when women smoked in their bedrooms with the transoms closed down and the windows opened wide." All the tobacco shops visited by the reporter agreed the number of female patrons they received had increased noticeably. At an exclusive Fifth Avenue shop the clerk said, "Oh, yes; a very great and noticeable increase. I think I might truthfully say that today 50 per cent of our patrons are women. They insist upon getting the same kind as the men." He also noted that because of more business from females his store had to carry more women smokers' supplies, such as cigarette holders, and cases. At another store a clerk commented that most of the increase in women smoking was due more to the fact that they were doing it openly than to anything else. "They've always done it, but it's been under cover. If they're going to smoke they might as well be frank about it."[40]

Clara Savage, another reporter, did a similar tour of New York tobacco dealers a year later, in 1921. Explaining the increase, a cigarette manufac-

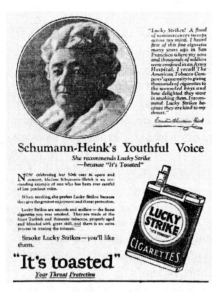

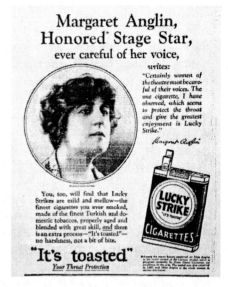

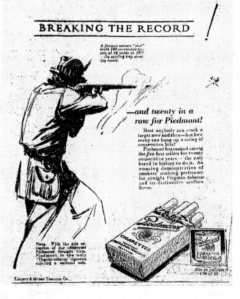

Top left: This 1927 endorsement ad was allegedly phony. Such embellishments by tobacco makers were not rare. *Top right:* Endorsement ads by women smokers began in 1927 and remained popular for decades. *Right:* This 1927 ad talked of a famous woman shot, but did not name her.

turer/dealer told her, "If a person lives in a town or even a medium-sized city he probably doesn't see many women smoking. They smoke in secret. He should have a look at our books and see what a tremendous mail order business we do with women." According to him they did not want to personally buy cigarettes in their own small communities, as they did not want their next-door neighbor to know they smoked. "When they send in their order for several hundred cigarettes— we do not sell less than a hundred— they ask us to send them in plain wrappers." All the tobacco shop personnel she spoke to told Savage that New York women were not among the secret smokers but had come out into the open about cigarettes. Remarked one shopkeeper, "They come into the store and buy their own. They used to send their husband or their brothers or someone else's brother, but now I should say that half of my customers are women." Among the reasons given for the increase were the influence of European women, the greater freedom of females, and changing fashions.[41]

Harry Burke was another journalist who explored the prevalence of the habit, writing in the *Ladies Home Journal* in 1922. He said that various reasons had been given for the tremendous growth in the number of female smokers. "One set charges it to the general emancipation and freedom allotted to the fair sex in recent years. Another blames the stage and the movies, where women are shown in the midst of luxury puffing away at their cigarettes." According to him, the cigarette manufacturers denied that any lure was offered to women; on the contrary, they argued, the increasing number of women smok-

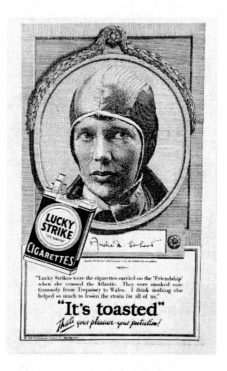

Note the somewhat subtle nature of this 1928 ad. A casual glance might have led someone to think famed aviator Amelia Earhart smoked Luckies. She was not a smoker. However, her male crew did indulge.

ers was a source of alarm. That was because female smokers were bound to increase the agitation against cigarettes and the manufacturers had their hands full counteracting the moves of reformers. Burke said there was still more smoking among the society set than among any other class in America, except perhaps the theatrical set. Also, Burke pointed to the number of Fifth Avenue jewelers who had departments devoted to handling cigarette accessories for women; with the more expensive places retailing cigarette holders for women at $50 to $500, with cigarette cases going from $50 to $1,000. Recently opened in New York was a unique store that was a combination shop and lounging room for the exclusive use of women smokers. An announcement card for that outlet declared, "The Advent of the Tobacco Shop, Catering to the Refined and Exacting Feminine Taste." The woman who managed that shop told Burke they had everything a woman required in the way of an accessory to her smoking, and the lounge

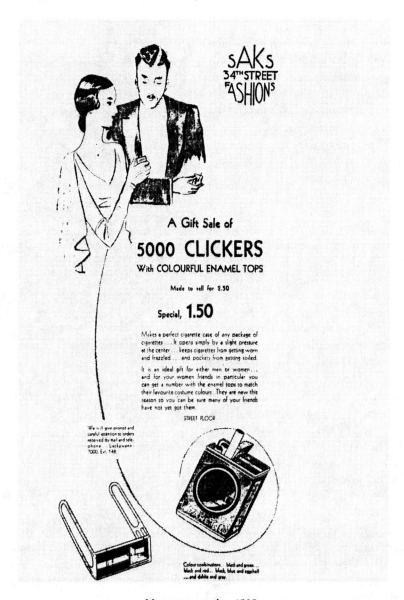

More accessories, 1929.

allowed them to smoke their brands "in repose." Color matching was also a feature of the shop, she explained. "If a woman comes in wearing a black costume we give her a black holder with a black silk-tipped cigarette." Additionally, the store provided hostesses with take-away cigarette arrangements for home use for that busy party planner. "The holders are in ten colors and made either of hand-blown glass or tortoise shell, and the cigarettes are silk tipped and in ten different colors. They are passed among the women on a silver tray and each selects the color harmonizing with her costume of the evening," she explained about the arrangements. Burke concluded, "Ten years ago the only cigarettes made for women were small gold-tipped, scented samples, about an eighth of an inch in thickness and two inches long. There is no demand for them today. Perfumed cigarettes are being made, but in the sizes used by men.... The perfumed blends are usually consumed by beginners among women," who soon switched to using the same brands men consumed. As evidence of that Burke said the manufacture of such cigarettes had been static with no growth over the previous 10 years, despite the enormous increase in cigarette consumption in general.[42]

Lecturing to a class of summer students at New York University in 1924, Charles Gray Shaw, professor of philosophy, told his class that despite their short hair, short sleeves, and cigarettes, women were becoming more womanly every day. Shaw argued that women were more moral than men but without being ethical, because they arrived at moral results "instinctively," without appealing to any ethical code.[43]

In the opinion of an anonymous female reporter in the *Washington Post* in 1924, women smoked not because they especially liked it or that they thought it made them look dashing; they smoked because they wanted something to do with their hands. She cited women sitting around for hours in some room or other listening to and taking part in "boring conversations that are only made tolerable by some trifling simultaneous activity. But what is that activity to be? Modern taste rules out woolwork and fancy embroidery, because of the hideousness of their products. There remains the cigarette." Waxing eloquent, she asked her readers to consider the possibilities open to such a woman who flourishes a cigarette: "How it can sustain the impressive pause; how it can point an argument, or deprecatingly play for laughs while appearing to avoid self-conscious humor; what it can express of character, in the way it is carried to the lips, the length of time it remains there, the precise flicking, or depositing of the ash, and above all the length of time the smoke itself is held back." For this woman, the cleverly used cigarette was a devastating drawing-room weapon, a fact known to every woman. And the women were far more adept at utilizing the cigarette that way than were men, although she did not explain why that was true.[44]

When an editor with the *Washington Post* asked himself, in 1925, why women smoked, he never got around to answering the question, but he did conclude, "The days when a cigarette between the fingers of a woman carried a stigma and branded her as an adventuress have long since passed. There are still some persons who try to connect cigarettes and morals just as there remain opponents of theaters and dancing."[45]

Public Places

When government-built dormitories were created for women war workers in Washington, D.C., in World War I, some 1,500 females flocked to them as soon as they opened — wars generally produced housing shortages. By 1919, with the war over, some women congressional employees were allowed in as well as females employed as clerks, secretaries, and so forth, to members of the U.S. House and Senate. One controversy that arose involved cigarettes. Some of the women who lived in the dorms smoked in their rooms and in other parts of the premises. Complaints were lodged by some of the nonsmokers who wanted a no-smoking rule in the facility and wanted it enforced. Female smokers argued it was the right of any woman to smoke in a hotel or a boarding house, if she desired, and the dormitories were nothing but hotels. Said one of the war workers still lodging there, "If Congress admits that women have a right to vote, I'd like to see them stop us from smoking. If a woman wants to smoke she'll smoke. You might as well try to stop a volcano from smoking."[46]

J. J. Rosenthal, manager of the Woods Theatre in Chicago opened a smoking room for women in his venue at the beginning of 1920. It had a marble floor, soft rugs, leather chairs and lounges and also contained a "box of cigarettes"—free to patrons—at an estimated cost of $10,000. As to the reason why he did it, Rosenthal explained it was because "the women drove him to it." He had found women smoking all over the place in his venue, in the lobby, in the waiting rooms, and in the washrooms. Two years later Charles Dillingham installed in his Globe Theatre (New York City) what he called the first exclusive smoking room for women in a New York theater. In it, cigarettes were provided free for women who had run out or had forgotten to bring their own with them.[47]

So common had it become by 1923 for females to smoke in theaters that the editor of the *Wall Street Journal* wondered editorially if we wanted that woman in those facilities. Editor Metcalfe complained abut the women who went "into the already crowded theatre lobby between acts to smoke cigarettes in the company of the men who have swarmed out at the fall of the curtain.... As a rule the woman who smokes because she wants to is content to enjoy her indulgences in the rooms provided for that purpose in most modern theatres." Even worse, thought Metcalfe was that the police wouldn't stop them because there were no laws against the practice; the managers of the venues would not stop them because they left patrons to sort such things out themselves; the male theater-goers would not register any objections. "Men are notoriously cowards in the face of the self-asserting woman, and generally the woman who smokes in the lobby looks as though she would not be a pleasant person with whom to have a public controversy," he explained. "The fact that she does what she does is presumptive proof that she would not be averse to attracting even more attention to herself." Despite what he had written, Metcalfe went on to declare his piece was not a protest against women smoking, "even in public, as that question has already been settled, as usual, in favor of the women doing what they please." Snidely he observed that without female smokers, the rather full life of New York's restaurants would be robbed of one of its most amusing features "in the person of the woman who doesn't care or know how to smoke, either in private or public, conspicuously and awkwardly smoking just to show that she's a devil of a fellow." Even the ones who "knew" how to smoke he condemned for their public "exhibitions of over-expertness in the handling of their cigarettes and the methods of their exhalation." Metcalfe concluded the kind of women who then smoked in theater lobbies would probably continue to do so "as good taste and gentle manners do not enter into their scheme of things."[48]

As of May 1921, women were allowed to smoke in the New York Athletic Club. Behind closed doors and at the end of a debate that resounded through the halls, that question was settled at a special meeting called to deal with it. Only men were in attendance at the meeting and only men voted; 187 opted for smoking by women, 134 voted against the proposal. That meeting was called in response to a resolution signed by 50 members of the club calling on the organization to annul the ban that had relegated the use of cigarettes by female guests to puffing away in hidden corners after public smoking by females had been definitely banned. Signers of the petition believed that because it had become the custom of other social organizations to allow women to be their own judges on the question of taste involved, their own club should no longer attempt to act as a censor over the behavior of women. Female guests at the club were mainly the wives of numbers, who were only allowed to enter the facility on Sunday nights and on a few special occasions by invitation. Those in favor of removing the ban cited the custom of "all fashionable hotels" of permitting women to do as they chose in the matter and insisted women might as well be allowed to smoke at their social gatherings since they did it at home anyway. Opponents noted that the New York Athletic Club had not allowed women to smoke by permission there in the club's 50-year history and asked why the ban should be lifted now. Also, they criticized the habit as unhealthful, called it "unladylike" and stressed the bad effect the habit had on women to raise their children to be "ladies and gentlemen."[49]

According to journalist Helen Bullitt Lowry, writing in 1921, it was only within the previous year that all New York restaurants allowed smoking by women. The Claremont was said to be one of the last in the city to yield, finally permitting the practice in August 1919. Ten years earlier, said Lowry, only foreign visitors thought of smoking in New York hotels and restaurants but by 1921 New York women in such facilities were "smoking like a chimney."[50]

The question whether smoking rooms should be provided in girls' clubs, community houses and other places where young women lived was the main topic of discussion at a meeting in 1922 of the directors of 30 such clubs. Women attending represented club homes operated under the direction of such organizations as the YWCA, the YWHA, the Ladies Christian Union, the Community Club and the Clara de Hirsch Home for Working Girls. The meeting was the monthly round table under the auspices of the League to Promote Proper Housing for Girls. With opinion divided on the subject, no formal action was taken, although a consensus seemed to be that women should be left to exercise their right of personal liberty.[51]

Reporter Harry Burke was one of those in the media who mentioned, in 1922, that the numbers of smoking women were increasing "in legions," and that they smoked the same brands as men, passing up the mild and scented brands supposedly made just for them, although they may have started on them when they first turned to the habit. According to Burke all the leading hotels and dining rooms in all the cities of any size, "except in a few remote case" had been forced to surrender and then allowed women to smoke in their premises. And, he said, "It is not uncommon to see women atop the Fifth Avenue buses puffing away at their cigarettes. The theaters are opening smoking rooms for women, and during intermission it is no longer unusual to find women smoking in the lobbies or on the sidewalks with the men."[52]

Marguerite Harrison argued that smoking in the women's toilets had been given de facto recognition by the conductors on most Pullman trains by 1922, particularly in the West, where it was said to not be unusual to see women smoking in the club car with the men, but in the East there were still conductors "with Puritan prejudices." Harrison concluded there was a growing demand for women's smoking compartments because the female public wanted a place to lounge and smoke just as much as the male traveler. Some day, she predicted, "the railroads will wake up to the fact, and then we shall no longer have to take our smokes, perched on the

Good tobacco comes back into style. *Anything* was a smoke during the War. But particular people are outgrowing their old recklessness. Tactful hostesses turn to Marlboros.

. . . . why take chances with cheap cigarettes?

Marlboros are the cigarettes of successful men. And dainty women. Marlboros are made for those who can afford 20 cents for the best. You will like them.

Before safety razors, most men grew whiskers!

Before short skirts, most women wore cotton stockings!

Before Marlboros practically everybody smoked cheap cigarettes!

Think how much pleasanter life is today with smooth faces, silk stockings, and Ivory-tipped Marlboros.

Successful men — and smart women—naturally turn to Marlboros. A cigarette for those who can afford 20c for the best.

Plain or Ivory Tipped
No difference in price

Marlboro ads in 1929 started out with the claim of being the smoke of choice among successful men and dainty women. After a brief run it was changed, for a much longer run, to successful men and smart women.

washstand or the toilet shelf, and another of the disabilities of women will have to be removed."[53]

In response to Harrison's piece, a Miss Gulliver responded that it was not necessary for women to retire to the toilets for a smoke. "Unless a sign says plainly, 'No smoking here,' you may smoke anywhere at all you choose," explained Gulliver. "Nothing unpleasant will happen." She had personally smoked on trains all over the country, without being sanctioned.[54]

When a reporter asked train personnel about stories about women invading the smoking car on trains (to smoke) conductors told him there was no law against it but traditionally only males used the smoker cars. However, those conductors admitted it was becoming more common to see women smoking in the smoker carriages.[55]

Another reporter mentioned at the start of 1923 that people had not yet gotten used to mixed smokers. He detailed a train ride he had taken in a smoker car over the busy holiday season, from New York City to Philadelphia and then on to Atlantic City. There were 50 seats in the smoking compartment, arranged in two rows of 25, on each side of the car facing each other. As the train left New York that car was fully occupied, containing 10 women and 40 men, with all but 6 or 8 of the latter puffing away as the train departed; none of the women were then smoking, although three were chewing gum. Said the reporter, "None of the women had yet lighted a cigarette. There was something formal and awe-inspiring about that car with its twenty-five chairs ranged on either side facing each other. Perhaps none of them would dare to smoke.... Finally, one of the women lighted a cigarette." In reaction there was a great amount of staring at her by other occupants of the car. After she finished her cigarette she took out a second one — but did not light it. "She looked around that silent, watching car full of unsure people and put the cigarette back in its case," said the piece. "It was no use. It was like making love at a funeral — distinctly inappropriate." Concluding his account, the journalist declared, "It is being done, because railroads are opening their smoking cars to women, but it is not being done comfortably."[56]

George MacAdam penned a long, full-page rant in 1925 against feminism in general and women smoking on trains specifically. He grumbled that the smoking car was the last of the old masculine institutions that females had reached out for and said "'This, too, is mine....' Well, the battle's over boys. We're licked. Our last sanctuary is gone; women have invaded the smoking car."[57]

In July 1925, what was said to be the first public smoking benches for women placed outdoors in New England were installed at Paragon Park in Massachusetts. Placed in front of the bandstand at the park the benches each carried a sign that read: "Reserved For Ladies (Smoking Permitted)." Installation was authorized by David Stone, head of the South Shore Amusement Park, after a "close study of the feminine demands of the present day." That study followed a dozen or more requests for such smoking benches that had been made at the Paragon Park administration office by women young and old.[58]

As of July 1925, women were allowed to smoke on the Detroit street railway lines. Hugh Wallace, general manager of the municipally owned local transportation system ruled in favor of the practice after receiving an opinion from the city's Corporation Counsel that it would not violate any city ordinance. Wallace's order said that smoking by women would be allowed on rear sections of trailer cars—where men were already allowed to puff. Frank J. Denney, Wallace's chief assistant, explained the decision by saying, "There is no law in the State of Michigan that prevents women from smoking. If they want to smoke and the privilege is extended to men, there is no reason why they should not be permitted to do so."[59]

Commenting on Wallace's decision, an editor with the New York Times was moved to remark that it represented another advance by smoking women. But he noted one remaining taboo, "As yet women do not smoke in the street — it would be interesting to know just why. But now in Detroit they permit women to smoke on open cars. One short step and the sidewalk also will be achieved by the touch of feminine progress." He went on to predict a future "where women have conquered so much they may yet walk the streets smoking cigarettes in long pants."[60]

Meanwhile in Chicago, after years of requests to women that they not smoke, one of Chicago's oldest and most famous restaurants, Henrici's, finally yielded in 1927 and allowed its women patrons to smoke. Reportedly it was the last restaurant in downtown Chicago to succumb. Permission for women to smoke was extended experimentally at first, to take care of the demands of theater crowds from 9 p.m. until midnight. "Then the demand for the raising of all bars became so strong that women at last may smoke at breakfast, luncheon, dinner or supper," explained the story. "Men always have been permitted to smoke at all hours."[61]

As noted, street smoking was the last remaining taboo for the females who smoked. A few women did breach that social convention but for those who did it remained, throughout this period, a behavior pattern likely to cause problems for those who indulged. In Kansas City, Missouri, on September 7, 1920, a woman asked police officer W. H. Scott, on the street, how to reach an address. Scott told her. "Thanks," said the woman, and reaching into a pocket of her coat took out a plug of tobacco and bit off a chew. Scott then arrested her on a charge of disturbing the peace. In municipal court on September 8, Judge John M. Kennedy dismissed the charge against her, by noting, "If women may vote, why shouldn't they chew."[62]

Edna Hobbs, 18, of Flatbush Avenue, Brooklyn, was arrested in July 1922 for smoking cigarettes in the street. Arraigned in Police Court, she was found guilty on a charge of disorderly conduct. However, on her appeal County Judge McLaughlin of Brooklyn overturned the earlier ruling when he decided that Hobbs had committed no crime by smoking in the street.[63]

About a month later Mary Sladden, 19, was walking along the street with her husband at Eighth Avenue and Twenty-Eight Street in Manhattan smoking a cigarette. Policeman Peter Kilyon reportedly "sharply" ordered her to throw away that cigarette. When she failed to comply, the officer allegedly knocked the cigarette from her hand by rapping her on the knuckles with his nightstick. When asked to comment on a report that Kilyon would be brought before him because of the incident, Police Commissioner Enright stated, "I have received no official notice of the episode and have no comment to make on it unofficially." After interviewing a number of police officers, a reporter said several thought an officer would exceed his authority if he ordered a woman to stop smoking as there did not appear to be a law covering such a situation. However, others thought it was largely a matter of the officer's discretion; all agreed it opened an ambiguous subject with many gray areas.[64]

In May 1926, a woman was fined $5 and 14 men were fined $3 each by Magistrate Edward Weil in New York with all of them charged with committing the same offense a day earlier — smoking on a Classon Point ferry boat. The 15 were arraigned on summonses charging them with a violation of the Sanitary Code in smoking in automobiles on a ferryboat. After the 14 men had been fined one by one, Virginia Barnes, 24, was called forth. On admitting the offense Weil fined her $5. "The extra two is for having the nerve to do it," he explained to her.[65]

Smoking a cigarette in the street in Greenwich Village, New York, resulted in a night in jail in the summer of 1926 for Mayonne Bayer, a 21-year-old schoolteacher, and her companion, Lewis Resnick, 24. They were arrested shortly after midnight at Third Street near Greene Street by police officer Henry J. Olsen, who took them to the police station on a charge of disorderly conduct. According to their story, as they walked toward a subway station Bayer lit up a smoke; Resnick was already smoking a cigarette. Suddenly out of the darkness came a commanding voice, "Drop that cigarette," and the policeman appeared. Bayer said the officer told her it was not a crime to smoke on the streets but "it wasn't nice." An argument ensued and the pair was taken to the station house. Olsen stated the pair had become boisterous— something they denied. Arraigned the next morning in court before Magistrate August Dreyer, all charges against the couple were dismissed.[66]

Police Magistrate Louis I. Turner held in court in June 1927 in Asbury Park, New Jersey, that asking a woman for a cigarette in the street was not sufficient grounds for having a youth arrested on a charge of disorderly conduct. Samuel Fried, 20, had been arrested on that charge on a complaint brought by Julia Faulhaber. Turner told the complainant that "many dignified, respectable women" smoked and that Fried was not presuming too much when he merely asked her for a cigarette.[67]

Medical Opinion

Medical advice offered in this period regarding women and smoking was always negative, albeit sometimes weird. A story datelined Paris in 1921 said that beards and mustaches were increasing "alarmingly" among women year by year with doctors blaming mainly cigarette smoking and alcohol drinking for the phenomenon. Statistics from the hospitals were said to show 11 percent of female patients to have an "abnormal" growth of hair on the upper lips and chins, whereas 27 percent of female inmates in the insane asylums were bearded or had moustaches. Paris society women, having taken up "intensive" smoking along with adopting the cocktail habit were said to be "aghast" over statements by leading Paris medical personnel that tobacco and alcohol were conducive to the development of unsightly hair. Physicians and beauty specialists in the United States, though, were quick to ridicule the idea of beards arising from smoking or drinking.[68]

An unnamed British physician declared in 1922 that the enormous increase in cigarette smoking among women called for some protest from the medical profession because the habit in many cases had passed "beyond a pleasure and become a vice." The absorption of nicotine, he explained, produced a condition of nervous distress that could become quite severe. In fact, the damage could be so severe as to cause mental instability. "Woman's delicate nervous organism was certainly not intended to endure large doses of this poison," he explained. "Her functions as a mother cannot but be interfered with when she indulges to excess."[69]

Journalist Harry Burke said in 1922 that medical men conceded that cigarette smoking in moderation was not injurious to the average man, because his vitality, his outdoor life, and the opportunity he had for exercise offset the injurious effect of the nicotine he inhaled. But there was no such counteracting influence in the case of females, he submitted. Women were not inclined to be moderate, and their habits of life accentuated the danger and the injury resulting from excessive smoking. Burke declared that while there was a divergence of opinion among medical men regarding the danger from nicotine to men if inhaled to excess, "there is one question upon which there is the fullest accord: Cigarette smoking is injurious to women; it induces increased pulse rates, heightened blood pressure and irritable hearts." Dr. Samuel Lambert, physician to Theodore Roosevelt, was cited as saying cigarette smoking among women was intolerable and a menace to their health. Burke believed women who smoked cigarettes could not be moderate in the habit. "At best it is a horrible weed and should be let alone. It fouls the breath and makes women unwomanly." Dr. Samuel A. Brown, chief of Bellevue Hospital in New York, argued smoking was much more injurious to women than to men. "Cigarette smoking in excess decreased the muscle activity and vitality and is very objectionable," explained Brown. "Men take more exercise than women, and the effect is not so noticeable or injurious. Women who smoke cigarettes usually sit around, ride about in their motors, attend teas, dinners or social affairs and get very little real exercise. Their mode of life is entirely different from that of men." Brown added that women smoked nervously

and could not smoke moderately. "From the standpoint of health, cigarette smoking among women is very objectionable and, on the other hand,
it is a let-down of moral standards."[70]

Antoinette Donnelly, a reporter, wrote in 1924 about the recent case
of a 23-year-old society girl in Boston who had committed suicide and
whose father attributed the act to his daughter's weakened physical condition that he said was due to cigarette smoking and the swift social pace
she was following. Donnelly said that story had stirred up a minor flurry
of protest against the woman with the nicotine habit. Admitting that many
observers had argued the role of the cigarette in the girl's death had been
exaggerated, she nevertheless said that if a constitution was not strong
then nicotine played havoc with the lungs, digestion and mucous mem-
branes. She then interviewed a number of medical people, all of who
pointed out negative effects of smoking. Dr. I. W. Vorhees of the Manhattan Eye, Ear and Throat Hospital, said, "In women, because she is more
highly sensitized than men, tobacco reacts more unhealthfully on the system." One unidentified physician felt that up to a certain point the criticism against cigarettes for women was "an esthetic thing," pointing out
that large numbers of women smoked in various parts of Europe and had
done so for a long time, with the result that people were used to that and
took little notice. In America, though, it was still a newer and less prevalent habit. Donnelly then moved on to attack the practice on moral
grounds; "there remains the final charge against women that the habit is
not a dainty one.... The odor of tobacco gets into the hair and it clings to
the breath — and the more one smokes, the more marked is this distress-
ing feature." Donnelly concluded, "Daintiness is the charm de resistance —
the one form of feminine attractiveness upon which all men agree. Yellow
teeth, stained fingers and a tobacco scented breath are what's wrong with
the picture."[71]

Medical attacks on women who smoked also emphasized more and
more the detrimental effects the habit had on beauty. Viennese physician
Dr. R. Hofstatter declared in 1924 that women who were heavy smokers
lost their fair complexions much more quickly than did nonsmoking
women. The facial features of the smoking woman, he contended, were
usually much "sharper" than those of nonsmokers; "The more women
smoke, the sharper the nose and chin are outlined. The skin becomes taut,
the lips lose their rosy color and become pale, while the corners of the lips
show wrinkles prematurely."[72]

Holding similar views was Dr. Cecil Webb-Johnson, one of England's
best-known specialists on diet and obesity, and author of a book on beauty
and women. He felt that tobacco use by women had a tendency to destroy

their "daintiness." As well, he subscribed to the idea women had trouble in being moderate in many areas. "A man often will have his allotted daily ration of so many pipes, cigars or cigarettes, but a woman is more unstable and less capable of self-control," he asserted. And, as a rule, he added, "a woman smoker does not appear to know what moderation means, any more than a woman drinker." Concerning the effects of excessive cigarette smoking upon a woman's beauty, Webb Johnson said, "Observe a girl who smokes excessively, and you will notice that she also looks undernourished, with staring eyes and a yellowish skin. To make matters worse, the smoke-dried throat experiences a false thirst, and thus more liquid than is necessary is consumed and an alcohol habit set up. The cocktail and the cigarette always go together."[73]

At a convention of beauty shop operators in New York in 1926, Joseph Byrne, managing director of the National Beauty Shop, said that women, if they continued to smoke, would soon look like men; the tobacco face was becoming more common among women. He then went on to give a description of a tobacco face that matched almost word for word that attributed to Dr. Hofstatter, with the addition that "the lower lips show a tendency to project beyond the upper lips. The eyes acquire a stare and the lids rise and fall more slowly."[74]

Dr. Joseph C. Bloodgood of Johns Hopkins medical faculty in Baltimore warned women they should not undertake any weight-reducing measures without first consulting their physicians to see that they were medically sound and the dieting measure was not quackery. He said, "Especially dangerous is the habit of smoking cigarettes for the specific purpose of cutting down the appetite and thus reducing weight. Undoubtedly many women are doing that now."[75]

In 1926 when a man named C. H. Kimball saw a report purporting to claim Dr. W. J. Mayo had stated his approval of smoking by women he wrote to the famed doctor. Mayo's secretary, Nora A. Guthrey, sent him a reply in which she said Mayo had been cited out of context. She said, in part, "I happen to know that Dr. Mayo has never smoked and that no woman member of his family smokes. I have heard him say, many times, that he is sufficiently old-fashioned to dislike to see women smoke; that admitting that a woman has as much right to smoke as a man, his sense of justice would make it difficult for him to vote against it, and he would dislike to vote for it."[76]

A warning to female smokers was given in 1926 by Dr. Herman Prinz, professor of pathology at the University of Pennsylvania, when he spoke at a convention of the Dental Society of the State of New York. With the increase in the number of women smokers, said Prinz, there was a grave

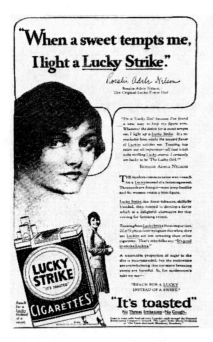
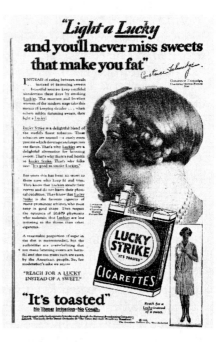

Left: How to stay slim — take up smoking, 1929. *Right:* Another one of Lucky Strike's 1929 stay slim (highly controversial) ads.

danger of cancer such as women of the Orient — who were heavy smokers — reportedly experienced. Prinz said that in the Orient the deaths from cancer among women were much greater than among men, and an overwhelming majority of those deaths were traceable to mouth diseases caused by the use of tobacco. According to statistics, stated Prinz, "50 percent of the cancer cases in the U.S. were due to buccalleucoolakia, which started on the tongue, and was the most common mouth disease caused by tobacco."[77]

Austrian ear, nose and throat specialist Dr. Franz Fremel said, "Smoking isn't doing women any good, it enlarges their vocal cords, makes their voices harsh and guttural, instead of soft and sweet, and creates a general catarrhal condition." Next to dust, he said, smoking caused the most throat trouble.[78]

On the occasion of her 50th year in the practice of medicine, in 1926, Dr. Eliza Mosher — one of the foremost women physicians in America — said she felt smoking was no worse for women (except during pregnancy and nursing) than it was for men, and that smoking both for men and women was without doubt injurious except in extreme moderation. She also mentioned the dangers of passive smoking for children.[79]

11

The Opposition, 1919–1927

"Threats of prohibition of tobacco have aroused the traders and workers to action. We are not going to sit idly by and see a wonderful industry destroyed by meddling women who have no conception of the problem they are attempting to solve."
— P. H. McCartin, Tobacco League, 1919

"If American women are to be leaders of the women of the world they must keep themselves without taint, and that includes the smoking of cigarettes."
— Mrs. John Henry Hammond, 1922

"Of course, the cheap sheik sport will encourage the flapper to smoke.... Yet I think not one real man in 100 can or does vision his wife with a little babe at her breast while smoking and spitting over its head."
— E. D. Goode, 1925

The opposition to women smoking in this period remained very strong, very vocal, very unsuccessful, and often very weird. A 1919 account claimed that an association opposed to national prohibition surprised some prohibitionists in preparations for a campaign to secure the prohibition of tobacco smoking following the prohibition of the sale of alcohol. (The 18th Amendment to the U.S. Constitution, Prohibition, was ratified by the states in 1919 and remained the law of the land until 1933 when the 21st Amendment to the Constitution, the repeal of the 18th Amendment, was ratified by the states. Ratification and then enactment of Prohibition gave a big psychological impetus to smoking opponents to continue the fight.) That group made public extracts from what it described as the textbook of the new antitobacco movement. Written by Professor Roman of Syracuse University *Nicotine Next* made the argument that smoking was harmful to morals. One part of the tract was an appeal to females employed at cigarette counters and shops to give up the work because it was conducive to immorality. Wrote Roman, "Go to any hotel, you will find the cigarette girl subjected to the same form of humiliation and insult that her sister barmaid formerly endured.... There should be a law in every State forbidding women to sell tobacco on the ground that it jeopardizes morals."[1]

The increased use of tobacco among women during 1919 was "appalling," according to the board of Temperance, Prohibition and Morals of the Methodist Episcopal Church. In a statement the Board made an earnest appeal to women to refrain from the use of tobacco "in the name of the country's welfare." No nation could maintain the vigor that had been characteristic of the American people after its women began the use of cigarettes, the statement warned. "The sedentary life of women tends to an excess in the use of tobacco and produces more serious results than is caused by its use among men. The nervous constitution of a woman has been compared to that of an adolescent boy. The effect of tobacco upon women is similar to its effects on immature youths," continued the advice.[2]

From its headquarters in Washington, D.C., the Methodist Episcopal Church condemned female smokers as a menace to the nation. Admitting there was justice in the demands of feminism that women be granted every privilege that men were entitled to, the church made the point that equality could not be granted in smoking because "the most serious factor, however, is the innate physical difference between men and women, involving a difference in responsibilities, a difference in duties and privileges. The woman at regular periods suffers nervous disturbances." And, continued the warning, "At the time of change of life, the woman is nervously unstrung, sometimes to the point of insanity. If she uses tobacco at this time her health is seriously handicapped."[3]

So extreme was the Methodist admonition against smoking that it brought forth a reply from the Federation of Women's Clubs. Frances Yawger, a past president of that group, responded that the matter of smoking was nobody's business but that of the individual woman concerned. "If smoking is a menace to the health of women, I believe women can be trusted to know it," she remarked. "No woman is going to allow anything to interfere with her health or the welfare of her children that the reformers are always scolding her about."[4]

A few months later, at its 1920 convention in Des Moines, Iowa, the use of tobacco by women was condemned by the General Federation of Women's Clubs. Adopted at the gathering was a resolution that the cigarette habit was increasing among women and that the use of tobacco was harmful to them.[5]

Regarding that resolution, an editorial in the *New York Times* commented that the practice was one regarded as objectionable by many people "but this objection is on the ground of taste, not of morality — it is, at any rate, if the people objecting are wise as well as estimable." Still, the editor thought the clubwomen's discussion and resolution on the issue was all too trivial and a waste of time. "Surely there are enough things of real importance crying for consideration these days, and the clubwomen cannot for a moment believe that their condemnation of the cigarette will have any reformative weight or effect on or out of club."[6]

Preaching before the congregation of the Free Synagogue in New York in 1921, Rabbi Stephen S. Wise condemned smoking by women, drinking by young people, lewd dancing, seminude dressing, attendance at all-night parties, and the use of lipstick. He argued that women were making a terrible mistake in "lowering" their standards to the level of men's. Much of the blame for the situation was attributed by Wise to the Europeanization of American standards. "The action of women with regard to freedom, who think that the only sure tokens of women's freedom are to be found in illimitable indulgence in smoking and drinking makes one wonder whether their emancipation came centuries too soon or a century too late," he complained. "To confound disgusting habits with independence is a strangely perverse attitude of mind."[7]

In an attack on the antismoking movement, the *New York Times* editorialized that it was well known to students of pioneer history that many grandmothers then smoked — not cigarettes but corncob pipes— and they were the pioneers that made America what it was. The editor added that a generation or two intervened in which grandmothers did not smoke anything, between the demise of the pipe and the rise of the cigarette. "But it is sadly characteristic of the moralist as he nowadays flourishes that he instinctively abandons the solid ground of his cause and wages war against the shadow of a name. He attacks not drunkenness, but all uses of beverages; not narcotic poisoning, but all use of cigarettes," commented the editor. "It would quite possibly mark an advance if both men and women were to give up cigarettes altogether. But if so it must be of their own will and judgment, not as a result of the beating of tom-toms, the imposition of a taboo."[8]

Mrs. William Atherton Du Puy, national president of the League of American Pen Women (it had 5,000 members) addressed the New York branch of the league in 1921. Her ire had been aroused by an article written by Elinor Glyn in *Cosmopolitan* that was highly critical of the modern American girl. Glyn attacked the American girl for wearing too few clothes, being lazy, not studying, having no religion, and so on, and declared flatly that no man would marry the "cigarette smoking, senseless American girl of today." Du Puy called the piece "a vicious attack" and remarked, about Glyn's charge, "Yes girls do smoke, and there is no harm if they don't go to excess."[9] Around the same time, meeting in Philadelphia, the National Council of Women passed a resolution urging legislation that would prohibit the sale of cigarettes to women.[10]

Cigarette smoking by women was condemned in 1922 by Bishop A. S. Lloyd of New York and Mrs. John Henry Hammond at a meeting of the Castle School alumnae in New York. "If American women are to be leaders of the women of the world they must keep themselves without taint, and that includes the smoking of cigarettes," explained Hammond. Lloyd said he agreed with her and when he compared European women with American women one of his reasons for preferring the latter was that cigarette smoking was not as prevalent in the United States among women.[11]

Four hundred members of the Albuquerque, New Mexico, High School Girls' League went on a reformist tear that same year and banned jazz dancing, petting parties, and cigarette smoking. Jazz dancing was described in a resolution as "dancing that involves unnecessary bodily contact and that might appear vulgar to the onlooker."[12]

At a meeting held near Chicago in May 1922, war on smoking among women was declared by four organizations devoted to the antitobacco crusade. Those groups hoped to unite into a single organization but never did. In attendance were representatives of the Anti-Cigarette League, the No-Tobacco League of America, the Narcotic Abstinence organization, and the No-Tobacco Army.[13]

Greenwich Village in New York had a reputation in the 1920s of attracting artists, writers, painters, creative types, Bohemians, and so forth, to live and work within its confines. Speaking at a dinner of the Neighborhood Council of Greenwich House, Municipal Court Justice William J. A. Caffrey criticized those types of people for lowering the neighborhood and good name of the Ninth Ward (it contained Greenwich Village). No amount of intellectuality would atone for the condition of those "unconservative" people, he warned. The fact that intellectuality stood out in certain quarters meant nothing because, Caffrey said, "What we want is a safe, sound conservative type of the average man and woman. We have got to fight for it so that the very foundation of the old Ninth Ward will not crumble." With regard to the neighborhood being treated as a curiosity he warned, "it will grow worse and worse so long as it permits women walking through the streets to smoke cigarettes." So shocking was the situation that he worried some of his listeners might not believe him, but he insisted it was a common sight to see women smoking on the streets "even in daylight."[14]

"If I could stop cigarette smoking in West Virginia I would consider it the greatest thing I could do for my State," declared Governor E. F. Morgan in 1924, commenting on the suicide of Margaret Harding in Boston. Specifically, the governor referred to a statement by the girl's father that attributed that suicide to cigarette smoking, among other things. Calling Mr. Harding's declaration as to the cause of his daughter's death "very courageous" and a warning to others, Morgan added he felt cigarette smoking among women was becoming "alarming" and he thought it was time the women's clubs took an active part in a campaign to stop the practice. Governor Morgan pointed out he had recommended bills to the last legislature that would have banned smoking cigarettes in public buildings, but those were not passed. "You cannot legislate morals into people," he observed. "You've got to preach it into them. That's why I think the women's clubs should take up the fight."[15]

Journalist Mildred Holland argued the smoking habit caused one to wear almost exactly the same "dreamy, sleepy expression" for as many minutes as one smoked and that the average person looked far less alert when smoking than when not indulging. A smoking woman on the stage, she felt, might look interesting and attractive for a few moments but no longer. And there were few (if any), instances of an actress on stage or screen smoking for more than a minute or two. That was because no professional director would allow an actress to limit the variety of her poses and expressions in the way that smoking made necessary. An actress on stage or screen might hold a cigarette in her hand a good deal, but, Holland commented, it was allowed to interfere with and partly hide the expression of her face only a fraction of the time. Regarding females who smoked, in general, Holland declared, "Any woman who smokes for more than a few moments is less interesting to look at than she would be if she were not continuing to smoke. Her ideas do not come as quickly; her face does not change as often; her whole manner and appearance change hardly at all." As another conclusion, she declared, "A smoking woman limits the infinite variety which is one of the basic principles of charm."[16]

Famed scientist Luther Burbank said in 1924 that he did not want to have anything to do with any woman who smoked, much less any clubwoman who indulged. The reason was that he looked to the females to lead in all moral issues and because he considered tobacco as bad for the constitution as morphine or any other deadly drug. Burbank wanted the clubwomen to start a crusade against nicotine; a campaign he felt should target not just women smokers but males also. "Tobacco kills," declared the plant specialist. "Smokers do not all drop dead around the cigarette lighter in tobacco stores. They go away, and years later, die of something else." He added, "I hope women will make war on tobacco because we shall have better health, more happiness, longer life and more comforts when we cease wasting our money for tobacco and whisky."[17]

When he gave a New York City lecture in 1924, Eugene Lyman Fiske, medical director of the Life Extension Institute, said the current weak spot in the work of life extension were the young women between the ages of 17 and 32. In Fiske's opinion they did not show as good a health record as their brothers, and the sickness rate was higher among young women than it was among young men. Fiske recommended, "Young women must study more carefully their habits of living, must avoid such injurious indulgences as cigarette smoking, late hours and loss of sleep; must give attention to exercise, fresh air and properly balanced diet."[18]

"Unusual" was probably an understated way to describe the complaint against smoking women raised by the Reverend H. C. B. Roger, vicar of Churchill and Blakedown, Worcestershire, England. Smoking by women should not take place, he felt, while they were sitting on tombstones. Writing in the parish magazine, the vicar said many Churchill female parishioners were using graves for their lounge and remarked that the sight of women sitting on tombstones smoking cigarettes was somewhat out of the ordinary. "It came as a distinct shock to me. Smoking is not a sin, and sitting on tombs is a harmless, if morbid, relaxation, but the combined effect, to put it mildly, is scarcely seemly, if not positively irreverent."[19]

When the *Times* of London reported on the opposition to smoking movement in the United States, in 1925, it did so partly in a sarcastic and mocking tone, referring to the American antitobacco movement in general as the "Legions of Gloom." Described was a meeting held a year earlier in Illyria, Illinois, during which the No-Nicotine Alliance proposed "in all seriousness" to try and get enacted a Constitutional amendment that would prohibit the sale and consumption of tobacco, as Prohibition had done for alcohol. Lucy Page Gaston was referred to by the English account as the "Carry Nation of Nicotine." According to this account, any such proposed constitutional amendment had no chance whatever of ever passing the U.S. Congress, let alone being ratified by the states. That proposed 20th Amendment read as follows: "(1) The manufacture, sale, transportation, inhalation or otherwise consumption of cigars, cigarettes, pipe tobacco, cut plug and snuff is hereby prohibited. (2) The Congress and the several States shall have concurrent power to enforce this article by appropriate legislation, and to appoint enforcement offices in every community." The reporter argued that American public opinion had all along been prepared to treat the matter as a big joke except "for the uncomfortable reflection that the anti-saloon campaign, which was for so long ridiculed, was carried to a successful conclusion on the legal, if not the practical side. So public opinion remains apprehensive of any reforming move initiated by the Legions of Gloom."[20]

E. D. Goode wrote a 1925 opinion piece in which he condemned all smokers, male and female, but especially women. "It seems that women with all their boasted intuition would realize that in aping men's habits they are losing men's reverence and respect. We are sure this is true, that the more women dress like, look like and act like men the less men admire them," he explained. But, Goode went on to warn, "Of course, the cheap sheik sport will encourage the flapper to smoke, making her believe she is a jolly good fellow, yet I think not one real man in 100 can or does vision his wife with a little babe at her breast while smoking and spitting over its head."[21]

Mrs. John B. Henderson, described as one of the leaders of Washington society, who presided at many affairs held at her home, announced in 1925 that she would launch a campaign against immodest dress. It was a campaign said to have the support of many society leaders as well as the officers of several women's organizations, including the DAR, the National Congress of Parents and Teachers, and the General Federation of Women's Clubs. When Henderson announced her campaign, she decried the wearing of short skirts and denounced cigarette smoking by women.[22]

Henderson entertained Washington's diplomatic circle and was the widow of a U.S. senator from Missouri. She wanted to see skirts come down to the ankle (the fashionable flapper length of the time was just below the knee). With respect to the antismoking part of her campaign, her announcement said, in part, "That, in the interest of future public health and efficiency, we pray that the comparatively new fashion of cigarettes be abandoned, in that reserves from health capital, expended to save the living organism from perils of poison inevitably lead sooner or later to physical bankruptcy and race degeneracy."[23]

One day later, in reiterating her declaration of war against the wearing of short skirts and cigarette smoking by American women, Henderson said women of the smart sets (fashionable, upper-class leaders) were the worst offenders with regard to "immoral" dress styles and smoking habits "and if the leaders of the women of this country lose their concept of womanly virtue and modesty, to whom are we to look for example?" She wanted to see "the total abolition of smoking among women." However, she refused to be quoted concerning the habits of men, content to declare the reforms she wanted (skirts to the ankle and no smoking by women) were sufficient for the time being and that other reforms could come later.[24]

Los Angeles journalist Alma Whitaker returned in 1926 with another caustic, sarcastic piece in which she attacked those who would stop women smoking cigarettes. She claimed that many women, especially clubwomen, teachers, and so on, officially still denied they smoked but did indulge privately; "It is almost the only secret vice otherwise righteous women allow themselves now." With respect to current reformers, Whitaker argued it should be made perfectly clear to the antitobacco reformers that they should start their work on the men. "The men began this thing (which is so vile dirty, immoral, disgusting—for women!) ... So they should certainly be the first to quit. They are braver, more strong-minded, self-controlled—and, ever so much more logical—than women." Plus, if men quit first, she added, "it wouldn't be so hard on them because they would still be getting our smoke by proxy, just as we had to bask in theirs by proxy, in the days of yore. And they would get the smoking kisses instead of us..."[25]

Still prominent in the antismoking movement in this period was the WCTU. Late in 1919 the Association Opposed to National Prohibition organized the Allied Tobacco League of America. Created at Cincinnati, Ohio, the new group vowed to wage a "militant" campaign against the WCTU's fight for a constitutional amendment prohibiting the growth, sale and use of tobacco and planned to devote itself to the general interest of the tobacco industry. Membership was to include growers, leaf dealers, warehouse men, manufacturers, jobbers and retailers of tobacco products as well as consumers. In a statement the antiprohibition organization explained, as an example of the need for the league's work, that the WCTU had filed in Oregon an initiative petition making unlawful the sale, use or possession of cigarettes in that state after January 1, 1920. According to the statement, WCTU tactics included not going at first to where tobacco was grown but attempting to drive in an opening wedge in states like Nebraska, Iowa, Kansas, and Maine where people were less directly connected to the industry. The WCTU, it was alleged, was following the strategy of the Anti-Saloon League, in that it was trying to achieve success by going through the old-time Democratic and Republican political bosses to achieve its goals, rather than to the people directly. Also reported by the statement was that there was a female superintendent of schools in Kansas, and also a member of the WCTU, who had said she would not approve the appointment of any teacher who used tobacco. Concluded the Tobacco League; "What these reformers are booked to encounter is the voice of a people weary of fanaticism, heckled to the end of all patience, and determined at last to clean house."[26]

Just a few weeks later, the national WCTU held its annual convention in St. Louis, where it declared it would not abate in any way its efforts of the past to educate against the use of tobacco. However, it was made plain by the WCTU, as if it wished to rebut critics who regarded the group as too fanatical, that no program would be arranged or carried out looking to state or national legislation on the subject.

At the convention, a resolution favoring the procuring of legislation, and perhaps an amendment to the U.S. Constitution against the sale, manufacture or use of tobacco, was introduced by a WCTU member described as "radical" who sought to carry the fight into the camp of the tobacco industry, since Prohibition (alcohol) had become a fact. But that resolution was reported to have been snowed under by an avalanche of opposition. Following defeat of that resolution, it was announced that the future attitude of the WCTU would be the same as in the past on the tobacco question. That attitude was to be one of education and not legislation, and officials of the WCTU asked the press to make that plain to the public in view of the fact that it had been charged that the WCTU intended "going after" the "unholy weed" in the same way it had waged war on liquor. WCTU officials explained that misinformation had been put out by an organization that had backed liquor in its fight against Prohibition and had never been true at any time. The group did say it would see that the law with respect to prohibiting minors from buying cigarettes was enforced, but other than that "it has no legislative war to make on the tobacco business." Despite such assurances, the Allied Tobacco League of America kept on working. It announced that literature was being printed to combat the work of the WCTU and that speakers would soon tour the country. P. H. McCartin, St. Louis representative of the Tobacco League, stated, "Threats of prohibition of tobacco have aroused the traders and workers to action. We are not going to sit idly by and see a wonderful industry destroyed by meddling women who have no conception of the problem they are attempting to solve."[27]

Four months later, when a reporter did a piece on the increasing prevalence of female smokers, he asked the WCTU what its position was. Ella A. Boole, president of the New York State WCTU, repeated the stance from the convention and in speaking of that resolve (no legislation, only education) declared that she wanted it known above all that the WCTU did not intend to "interfere" with men who had already formed the tobacco habit. "Our efforts are not directed in that field at all," she explained. "Men have smoked for years. We are not taking it upon ourselves to tell them at this late day that it is not good for them. But we are interested in holding in check the spread of smoking among the youth of the country and the women of the country."[28]

Just one year later, strict observance of the Sabbath, prohibition of smoking by minors and by adults in public places and the creation of sentiment against allowing women to sell tobacco in any form were urged in literature sent out by the national WCTU. Said a reporter, "In spite of denials of officials of the W.C.T.U., that they intended to do anything more than prevent smoking by minors, the literature distributed by them disclosed other objects." Among aims listed in a pamphlet titled "Plan of work—1921," sent out by Helen G. H. Estelle, superintendent of the WCTU's department of antinarcotics, were the following: "Create public sentiment against girls and women selling tobacco in hotels, railway stations, theater lobbies and elsewhere," "Petition colleges and clubs to abandon entertainments known as smokers," and "Smoking in hotels and restaurants is objectionable to many. In a tactful way protest to the owners against the custom." As well, readers of the pamphlet were urged to request their state Board of Health to forbid smoking in markets and stores where foodstuffs were sold; "If impossible to get a State law, work for a city ordinance" and "Ask for a local ordinance forbidding smoking in polling and voting places."[29]

An ultimatum was sent to a Huntington Park, California, café proprietor in April 1923 by 200 prominent delegates of the Los Angeles County WCTU. It said, "Dear Sir: We regret that we cannot patronize your café but we disapprove of the sale of cigarettes and certain beverages which you offer your customers." That message was put together following a two-hour session conducted by the antinarcotics department of the WCTU led by Mary T. Runnels, superintendent of the department. During the discussion several members of the organization learned they had patronized a café that served cigarettes and near beer to customers. Members who had eaten there admitted their "mistake" and apologized at the meeting. On the ground that they had been ignorant of the policy of the café, those miscreant members were forgiven. Runnels also gave an illustrated address on the evils of tobacco and liquor and urged the WCTU to use every effort to combat it.[30]

Mrs. John Le Page, president of the Mount Vernon, New York, chapter of the WCTU said that women would not be permitted to smoke in public in Mount Vernon if tentative plans of that branch were put into effect — they weren't. Le Page explained the matter had been discussed by the branch members who had decided to make a drive against the practice. "We believe that if women insist upon smoking they should be compelled to do so in rooms provided for that purpose and not in public places," said Le Page.[31]

Reportedly, a "sensation" was caused on the floor of the Ohio WCTU convention in Steubenville when delegates tried to force through a motion condemning Queen Mary of England's attitude in favor of women smoking. Florence Richards, president of the Ohio WCTU, however, halted the discussion declaring, "We have enough cleaning house to do here in America."[32]

Although Nebraska, Iowa, Arkansas, and Tennessee repealed their bans on the sale of cigarettes after the war, the antismoking movement (with the WCTU as a prime participant) managed to achieve passage of two new state laws. One, a ban on cigarette sales passed by Idaho in 1921, was repealed almost immediately. The other, a ban on cigarette sales and public smoking, backed by the Mormon Church, was approved by the Utah legislature in 1921 but was not initially enforced. When Salt Lake County sheriff Benjamin R. Harris, who won election on a promise to take Utah's ban on public smoking seriously, staged a crackdown in 1923, arresting three prominent citizens (men) who had lit up in a restaurant, he provoked a storm of controversy. Faced with nationwide ridicule and open hostility from the state's citizens, the Utah legislature quickly legalized cigarette sales to adults and cut back sharply on the restrictions on smoking in public.[33]

Lucy Page Gaston and her league also continued the fight, but Gaston was soon exiled by her own organization and her own people as she degenerated into little more than a national joke. At war's end she continued her fight against the cigarette with the same zealotry as before, apparently unable or unwilling to accept that the cigarette and its image had changed dramatically. Returned soldiers were confirmed smokers; more women were taking up the habit. Also, more men turned in their cigar or pipe in favor of the cigarette. Several states, realizing their statutes prohibiting cigarette sales were habitually broken, repealed them. Gaston had all her work to do all over again. Yet she vowed to fight on as she neared 60 years of age. However, the old Carry Nation tactics of reform by hatchet (verbal if not literal) were no longer suitable or effective in the post–World War I world; a world that abused her or laughed her away as an eccentric at best, an irritating crank at worst. Understanding that new methods were in order, the International Anti-Cigarette League started to concentrate on scientific aspects of the subject and to limit its work to educating boys and girls. Aware that Gaston, using the old ways, did not fit in and only generated a number of lawsuits, she was asked to resign from the league. She did that on the last day of 1919, almost exactly 20 years after she had formed its predecessor. Then Gaston got stranger still.[34]

On January 1, 1920, Gaston announced her candidacy for president of the United States. Her platform was clean morals, clean food and fearless law enforcement. She had breakfasted with a man who told her that extensive adulteration was being practiced; hence her clean-food plank. Gaston's morality plank, she explained, would take in not just smoking but also burlesque shows, suggestive movies, extreme styles, and modern dancing. On the stage and screen she wanted "clean, sweet things," community singing instead of dancing, debating societies and spelling bees instead of cabarets. Within six months she withdrew from the presidential race. Apparently she threw her support to William Jennings Bryan, for, in July 1920, when the Prohibition Party nominated Bryan by acclamation at its national convention in Lincoln, Nebraska, Gaston was a delegate from Illinois. When Warren Harding (an overt cigarette smoker) was nominated for president, she gave up national politics as hopeless. Ousted from the International League, she organized a new one under the old name, the National Anti-Cigarette League. With "Save the Girl" as her slogan and "Abolition of the cigarette in America by 1925" as her goal, she took her war and herself into Kansas, still in 1920, which was one of the few states that still retained its statute that prohibited cigarette sales to adults, although this law was not enforced.[35]

Late in 1920 Gaston, then in Topeka, announced she had sent a letter to president-elect Harding asking him not to smoke cigarettes. Her letter concluded, "The United States has had no smoking President since McKinley. Roosevelt and Taft and Wilson all have clear records. Is not this a question of grave importance?"[36]

In a protest against Gaston's letter, a carton of cigarettes, purchased by contributions of 10 cents each from 19 Atchison, Kansas, men, was mailed to Harding. With the smokes was a letter from Carl Brown, leader of the group, explaining the gift was prompted by Gaston's letter urging him to not smoke. "We do not necessarily defend cigarettes but we want you to understand that we resent pernicious audacity on the part of a female who writes you such an insulting letter under a Kansas date line." And in response to that gift to Harding, Richard J. Hopkins, attorney general of Kansas, formally requested attorneys at Atchison and Shawnee Counties to investigate possible violations of the state anticigarette law and to commence prosecutions if evidence warranted that. Both the sale and the gift of cigarettes were illegal under the Kansas law.[37]

A few weeks later Gaston announced she had received a reply from president-elect Harding. "I think it is fine to save the youth of America from the tobacco habit," he replied. "I think, however, the movement ought to be carried out in perfect good faith and should be free from any kind of hypocrisy or deceit on the part of those who are giving it their earnest attention."[38]

Although she was representing her own organization (the National Anti-Cigarette League) while she was in Kansas, she also had some type of employment arrangement with the Kansas Anti-Cigarette League (part of the International League that had recently dismissed her) that paid some of her expenses and a salary. However, just a few days after announcing Harding's reply, the Kansas League stated it would no longer pay any of Gaston's bills or her salary; effectively they had also fired her. While her shrill and harsh manner and tactics may have been enough to get her terminated, the specific spur to dismissal was said to have started when Gaston announced that *Coffin Nails*, a magazine devoted to anticigarette concerns, would be published by her out of Topeka. The headquarters of the International League in Chicago refused to approve the proposed publication. Gaston's only response was to announce she would leave immediately for Iowa, to continue the fight.[39]

After an apparently brief sojourn in Iowa, she returned to Chicago, still head of her National League, to fight it out with her old organization, the scientifically minded International League. Her tactics became more bizarre and desperate. At the start of 1922 Gaston (described by a reporter as America's "most active anti-nicotine crusader") declared that at last the harmful element in cigarettes had been discovered. That harmful ingredient was, she said, "furfural," described as a "colorless, aromatic, volatile, oily compound, gradually darkening, which is formed by distilling bran, starch, sugar, etc., with sulfuric acid." It was said to be produced by the burning of glycerin, used in cigarette manufacturing. According to Gaston, the furfural in one cigarette provided the equivalent "kick" to that found in two ounces of whiskey. She went on to deplore the increasing use of cigarettes by girls. Furfural's discovery was not the result of any scientific work or research. Rather, it seemed to have been something that Gaston manufactured from her imagination.[40]

At a convention of the International Anti-Cigarette League at Los Angeles in 1923, one of the speakers was Mrs. Charles Gray, former head of the Parent-Teachers' Association. She told the delegates of some of the effects of cigarettes on women's morals; it caused a general breaking down of moral fiber; it caused marriage bonds to be held "frivolously" with some women believing that "when they are done with one husband they can walk on to the next one." Another speaker declared the war against the evil influences such as smoking that were said to dominate in the women's clubs might be waged successfully if Christian women should join those clubs. However, doubts were expressed by some delegates that Christian women could gain entry to those clubs and even if they did they might not possess the education necessary to combat the "sinister influences."[41]

The Utah anticigarette law mentioned earlier was the last of its kind, although North Dakota and Kansas kept their similar statutes on the books until they were repealed in 1925 and 1927, respectively. Neither of them had ever been seriously enforced. When she returned to Chicago, Gaston lived from hand to mouth, relying on whatever donations she could muster. Still, she continued to roam the streets of Chicago and hectored any boys she found smoking on the street; she irritated and harassed prominent female smokers, as well as her old group, the International League. Gaston welcomed all reporters, even though she knew they would write "funny" stories about her. They still sought her out, partly because of nonsense issues like furfural, which, of course, was a powerful incentive for a funny story. At the start of 1924 she met G. Henri di Ronchi, a French man just arrived in the United States, who brought to her aid a new zeal and some money. But it was all too late, for no sooner had she recruited this disciple than she walked in front of a trolley car and was struck down by it in January 1924 as she was leaving an anticigarette meeting. Never fully recovered from her injuries, she died in August that year of an unrelated cause. Ironically, she died of a condition often associated today with cigarette smoking — throat cancer. Gaston, of course, never touched the weed. She died with the hope that her work, left in the hands of di Ronchi, would be carried on to a successful conclusion. However, Gaston's National League staggered along under di Ronchi's direction for only a few months before it, too, expired. Around the time of her death, the U.S. produced more than 50 times as many cigarettes as in 1899, when Lucy Page Gaston formed her first anticigarette group.[42]

One well-publicized effort to pass an anticigarette law specifically targeting women came in 1921; it was a bill under which the women of Washington, D.C., would have to stop smoking in public, if U.S. representative Paul B. Johnson (Mississippi) had his way. The bill he offered in the U.S. House of Representatives in June that year stipulated that it "shall be unlawful for any hotel or restaurant keeper or any other firm or corporation engaged in any public business in the District of Columbia to permit any female person to smoke cigarettes in any public place" (cigars, pipes, and so on, were not mentioned). Violators of the measure (proprietors and the women puffers) would be fined $25 for the first offense and $100 for each subsequent offense. Johnson, who had never smoked in his life, explained, "Why, I was walking down the street the other day and I saw a young lady take a cigarette out of the hand of the young man she was walking with, and take a puff herself. You can go to any hotel in Washington, to public functions and to places after the shows and see women smoking cigarettes. It is worse than whisky." Worried that smoking by women was constantly increasing he added, "It is a bad thing and is going to contaminate the race. A woman who smokes, and nurses her child, transmits the evil effects of smoking." He was of the opinion that the regulation of smoking by women came under police power "and as is well known police powers are practically without limit." Johnson even argued that all those females who smoked did not want to indulge at all, "They smoke because those who are looked upon as leaders set the pace and they feel that they have to follow and they are in favor of this legislation." Continuing, Johnson elaborated, "There is too much smoking by women in Washington. And there are a great many women who would like to have it ended. Besides the men do not look with respect upon women who smoke. I have been assured that I will have a lot of support for the measure. I was brought up to reverence women, but I must confess my respect for women drops when I see them smoking."[43]

Though not a smoker himself, Johnson said he was not opposed to men smoking, if they did not indulge too heavily in it. Public places were defined in his bill as dining rooms, restaurants, cafés, cafeterias, theaters, passenger elevators, streetcars, passenger coaches, depots, railway waiting rooms, motors or other vehicles employed as commercial carriers, and even "any other public place where two or more persons are gathered together."[44]

Openly contemptuous of the proposal was an editorial in the *New York Times* wherein Johnson was mocked: "Day after day his nostrils and his heart were offended by women shamelessly puffing coffin nails in public" and "He sees dangerous crime stalking, as such crimes always do, in the capital."[45]

Journalist Helen Bullitt Lowry did a long commentary piece on the Johnson proposal, starting off by remarking, "Hardly a week passes but somebody has an idea for legislating more morals into us." For women smokers and nonsmokers, argued Lowry, the issue was political and not personal because "feminist persons consider any bill important which brings up the question of 'class legislation' and 'sex legislation' and the outworn fallacy that woman is a ward of the State and not a citizen — while feminine persons in the official walks of life refer to smoking as not a moral issue at all, but merely a matter of taste." Said Mary Towle, a nonsmoking assistant U.S. district attorney, "What possible moral code is involved? The important question brought to light is whether any sex legislation is possible."[46]

Dr. Katharine B. Davis, supervisor of the Bureau of Social Hygiene, also asserted the issue had nothing to do with morals. Rather, "I am inclined to think that the prejudice against women smoking is one of those

conventions grown rigid — although it probably had its start in the clinging vine days when it wasn't considered attractive for women to be mannish — and from that point somehow got mixed up in people's minds with
'fastness.'" As far as Davis was concerned, the only sex legislation that had
a right to differentiate between the sexes was where the matter of mater-
nity was concerned. And even there, such matters were to be addressed by
physicians, not politicians. Davis castigated Johnson for what she saw as
an attempt by the politician to impose small-town and rural Southern values on the people of a sophisticated big city. One who favored the measure was Carolyn Voton, sister of President Harding and a social worker
with the District of Columbia Police Department. She despaired of working any permanent "regeneration" in the character of a girl who refused
to sign and abide by an anticigarette pledge. "I can't believe anything they
say, or depend on them to do the right thing unless they will first renounce
cigarettes." Voton declared smoking a "perfectly vile and filthy habit."[47]

An editorial in the Los Angeles Times took no obvious position on the
Johnson bill but quoted from a letter sent to the congressman from a female
schoolteacher in Iowa. "This has been a man's world long enough and the
women are now ready and willing to regulate their own affairs as soon as
you leave it to us and spend your own time and efforts in raising your own
standard," it said, in part.[48]

At the hearing in Washington on the Johnson bill, held in July 1921,
some 25 women spoke publicly on the proposal; they opposed it by a count
of 24 to 1. Hearing Chairman Focht, of the District of Columbia Committee, which held the hearing, offered the women spectators present the
opportunity to smoke if they wished, but not even one availed herself of
the offer. Reportedly the room was filled with spectators, many of them
female secretaries and stenographers from the offices of the representatives. In making his case for his bill, Johnson told the hearing that smoking degraded women, that it injured their health and morals and had a bad
effect on their children. Typical of the 24 women who spoke publicly
against the bill was Mrs. C. E. Cassidy, wife of a U.S. Army colonel. She
had never smoked, she said, but stated she objected to having any group
of men telling her what she should or should not do. Then the Johnson
bill vanished, never to be heard from again.[49]

Other jurisdictions entertained similar thoughts. The female smoker
came under discussion in March 1922 in Boston before the Legislative
Committee on Legal Affairs. Massachusetts representative Shulman of
Dorchester, appearing for his bill to prohibit women from smoking in
hotels, declared that he offered his proposal to raise the standards of
women, to check immorality in future generations, and to promote pub-

lic health. If women wanted to smoke, Shulman thundered, let them do it in private. In his opinion the smoking habit of women had been brought to Boston by a handful of females who saw it in New York and thought it would be a society fad in Boston. W. W. David, a spokesman for hotel men, said he did not like to see women smoke, but he thought it was "preposterous" to put the onus on hotels to curtail the practice. Nils T. Kjellstrom, speaking on behalf of the Association for the Preservation of Personal Liberty, remarked that decent women did not smoke, but, "If women are prohibited from smoking, then the men will be, and finally we shall have our meals and our clothing regulated." Shulman's bill would have amended the state's hotel laws so as to make the proprietor liable to a $100 fine if a woman smoked at his establishment.[50]

Rising to the occasion, perhaps partly because New Yorkers were blamed for women smoking in Massachusetts, the *New York Times* delivered another scathing editorial, this time on the Shulman proposal. "Boston's reformers, having nothing else to do in a city so nearly perfect, have undertaken to stop smoking in public places ... a vile habit imported from New York, the flourishing garden of all iniquities." One person who appeared at the Massachusetts hearing suggested that tobacco must be equally bad for men and demanded its prohibition for both sexes, if one were to be deprived of the item. "He made no hit at all with the reformers," stated the editor. "Yet, of course, he was quite right, and why is it only in public places that women need to be saved from the evils of nicotine. If bad there, smoking must be worse at home, where the opportunity for indulgence in the vicious practice is so much more prolonged." Then the Shulman bill vanished, never to be heard from again.[51]

Even New York City was not immune from the desire to introduce such legislation. A resolution to prohibit women smoking in public places was introduced in the New York City Board of Aldermen on December 20, 1921, by Alderman Peter J. McGuinness of Greenpoint, Brooklyn. Similar ordinances had appeared there before and the Greenpoint alderman made no more progress with his proposal than had his predecessors as his resolution was referred to the Committee on General Welfare, effectively killing it. McGuinness explained he had introduced the measure because of many complaints from women all over the city who objected to entering places where women were smoking. The proposed ordinance, which provided for a fine of $5 to $25 and/or imprisonment of up to 10 days for violators, read, "no person, firm, partnership, corporation or association of whatever character, owning or controlling wither as proprietor or manager, any hotel, restaurant, place of public entertainment or other place of public resort in the City of New York in which people meet and congregate whether for purposes of refreshment or entertainment shall allow any female to smoke in any such place." Then the McGuinness bill vanished — only it *was* heard from again, sort of.[52]

Suddenly, three months later, it was announced that a city ordinance had been passed by the Board of Aldermen on March 14 and put into effect on the night of March 22. That announcement came as a surprise to the aldermen, the police, and the city in general. Murray Hulbert, president of the Board of Aldermen, said he was positive no such order had been passed, although McGuinness, the bill's author, insisted that New York mayor Hylan had signed it. Nevertheless, it was made the subject of a general order by Police Commissioner Enright and sent to every station in the city. As police officers assembled at their stations before going out on duty the night of March 22, the order was read to the men. Also, some police personnel were sent to carry the news into places where women met and smoked. Hulbert continued to insist no such ordinance had ever been passed or even brought forward to be debated and voted on, although he admitted he was not in attendance at the March 14 meeting. Enright's police order stated the ordinance was passed by the Board of Aldermen on March 14 and signed by the mayor on March 21. When a reporter looked at the City Record of March 16 (which contained the official report of the Board of Aldermen meeting on March 14) he found it contained no reference to the passage of the ordinance. McGuinness remained adamant the ordinance had passed — even when he was told that Alderman Collins and other councilors also could not remember it, and those men had been in attendance at the meeting. McGuinness was unable to explain the general memory loss.[53]

That ordinance was the second such bill he had introduced. The one from late 1921 had been filed, shelved and killed. When he introduced it again, early in 1922, he said that he, his wife and his sisters had been shocked to see women smoking in restaurants. "The morals of our young girls are menaced by this cigarette smoking," he explained. "I wish to stop this cigarette smoking in the restaurants of our city." Especially troubling to him was what he declared happened to young men who went into New York restaurants to find women smoking cigarettes. "What happens? The young fellows lose all respect for women and the next thing you know the young fellows, vampired [seduced] by these smoking women, desert their homes, their wives and children, rob their employers and even commit murder so that they can get money to lavish on these smoking women. It's all wrong and I say it's got to stop." Under the ordinance the offending female smoker was not guilty of any crime or subject to any punishment, only the management of the public place that had allowed her to smoke.

Mary Garret Hay, spokeswoman for the National Women's Party, complained, "If they are telling the women they must not smoke in public they should tell the men not to also. It is perfectly ridiculous.... It is an infringement of personal liberty, as well as discriminating against women."[54]

Just as suddenly, on March 28, Police Commissioner Enright rescinded the order. It had all been a mistake. McGuinness had reintroduced his resolution on January 24, 1922, and it was "filed" (that is, referred to committee to die) by a vote of 55 to 3 against it moving any further along toward enactment (the same thing that had happened to the resolution McGuinness had introduced in 1921). Clerk Dan McCoy was an assistant in the office of the city clerk, with 40 years of service. He found the resolution among his papers, and, thinking it had passed, sent it to police headquarters, which acted on it as though it were lawfully passed even though the necessary signature of City Clerk Michael J. Cruise was conspicuously absent. McCoy's chief task was to notify each city department affected when the Board of Aldermen adopted an ordinance. Or at least, that was the only version of the tale officially released. Then the McGuinness bill vanished, never to be seen again.[55]

While that was happening, the City Council of Chicago defeated on March 29, 1922, a proposed ordinance that would have prohibited women from smoking cigarettes in public. While the ordinance was being discussed, five women appeared in the council chamber gallery smoking cigarettes. They were ordered to stop — a rule prohibited smoking by anyone in the visitor's gallery. An amendment was offered during discussion to include cigars and pipes in the banned list for women, but was rejected. Then a "joker" amendment was introduced that provided it would be unlawful "for any female to appear in any public place wearing rolled stockings, skirts shorter than four inches above the ground, penciled eyebrows, bobbed hair unless enclosed in a hair net, galoshes unless buckled, or low-cut dresses unless approved by the city morals commission."[56]

The last law on the books of a jurisdiction that banned the sale of cigarettes to adults was found in the state of Kansas; it prohibited the sale, or gift, of cigarettes to anyone within the state. The state Senate of Kansas passed a bill repealing that law, by a margin of 26 to 9, in February 1925. In an understatement, a reporter suggested in the previous few years the statute had not been "rigidly enforced." Still, it took some more time before that law, enacted in 1909, was gone. Kansas governor Ben S. Paulen signed the repeal measure into law in February 1927. It was agreed that the only effect of that law in recent years had been to raise the retail price of a 15-cent pack of cigarettes (then the going rate in most of America) to 25 cents. Despite the law, they were retailed much like they were in states with no such law.[57]

By the end of this period, 1927, women had made large gains in terms of being allowed to smoke. Gone was the time when it was all done covertly. It had spread to many public places, well beyond restaurants and cafés. Also, the young, intellectual class of women had adopted the habit and practiced it in the halls of higher learning. Stigmatization of smoking women was much less common, but certainly not absent, and those who leveled such attacks were increasingly seen as the problem, more so than puffing females. Organized opposition to the habit stopped by around this time. Gaston was gone and her old group, the International League, and the WCTU would not be heard from again. Not that the opposition disappeared; it was limited more to isolated individuals or small weak groups. All those increases in the numbers of women smoking through to the end of 1927 were achieved without any push from advertising. Prior to 1927 there were virtually no tobacco ads that targeted women, directly or indirectly. All that changed in 1927 when advertising finally started to target women, perhaps not coincidentally to the repeal of that last anticigarette law in Kansas, in 1927. For the remainder of the innocent years, 1927 to 1950, the major issue of focus on women and cigarettes was in advertising. But advertising could not be blamed for the number of females who smoked by 1927; it played no part in their recruitment.

12

Abroad, 1927–1950

"The German woman does not smoke."
— Signs in Nazi Germany public places, 1933
"Every cigarette that female students do not smoke now saves one for the soldiers on the front."
— Anne Kothenhoff, Germany, 1940

In a somewhat unusual admission in France in 1928, the responsibility for the fact that many French women smoked was assumed by M. Blondeau, director general of the government Tobacco Service. He related how he undertook a few years earlier to find a way to induce women to become general consumers of tobacco and how he had succeeded. With the manufacture and sale of tobacco in France then a state monopoly, the results of his efforts contributed materially to the finances of the nation. "When I became Director of the Tobacco Service," explained Blondeau, "it occurred to me that if I could get the women to smoke I could bring about an important increase in the consumption of tobacco, and hence increase the profits to the state. It was an extensive undertaking." He added that he wanted to cultivate the "feminine taste" for light tobacco. Cigarettes then produced by the French state were said to have left a good deal to be desired. So they set about trying to improve them. "We succeeded, and now we have put on sale a whole series of light cigarettes of a high order," said Blondeau. "We have taken especial care to put them into attractive boxes. Women cannot resist a pretty box, whether it contains candy or cigarettes. They began to smoke and they have continued." As a result of his scheme, the consumption of cigarettes made of light tobacco by the state, which had been 50,000 kg annually before World War I, then was 300,000 kg. "We have not overlooked the element of salesmanship," he remarked. "Retailers have been encouraged to make a better display of cigarettes; so that today one may offer a pretty woman a box of cigarettes as appropriately as a box of chocolates."[1]

Later that year, France's first Smokers' Congress was held in Paris. One male delegate complained about the lack of courtesy he found in female smokers. In the old days, he said, before women became "incessant" smokers, it was customary for men to ask permission to smoke in railway carriages, restaurants, and other public places. But today, he thought, the nonsmokers had no refuge from the woman who smoked whenever and wherever she pleased and never asked permission.[2]

Several years later, in 1934, the Paris correspondent of the London *Daily Telegraph* wrote a piece in which he claimed French women almost never smoked in public. According to him, only about 2 percent of the women in France smoked at all, with most of those living in the cities. "In the French provinces it would never enter a woman's head to smoke," he added. "There is no smoking among Frenchwomen of the working classes, either; there has never been a campaign against women smoking as in Germany, for there has been no need for it."[3]

Britain's powerful cocoa cartel dominated the world's cocoa market for some years, only to collapse in 1928 and cease to function as a unified cartel because prices and profits had fallen to such a low level the trust could no longer operate. And women were blamed for it all, specifically women smokers. Women's substitution of cigarettes for chocolates, which was then making the fortunes of tobacco companies, had a reverse effect on members of the cocoa trust. One explanation put forward was that it went back to World War I when candy was hard to come by (sugar was rationed and candy sent to the troops) but cigarettes were said to have been plentiful and easier for women to obtain.[4]

English newspapers reported in 1930 that Queen Mary was a "regular cigarette smoker." According to the *Evening Standard* the news was not at all startling because

> long before smoking had ceased to be thought freakish or fast for the average Englishwoman, royal ladies having cosmopolitan ways smoked, as did their French and Russian cousins. Queen Alexandria smokes, so do her daughters, though naturally they would not be seen smoking on formal public occasions, and it will be remembered that cigarette cases which appeared among Princess Mary's wedding presents were not sent by complete strangers.

It was said that many females invited to royal banquets for the first time refrained from taking a cigarette after dinner for fear of displeasing Queen

Mary, only to be agreeably surprised later when the queen urged them to have a cigarette with her.[5]

In an editorial on Queen Mary being a regular smoker the *New York Times* thought the only portion of English society likely to be upset by the news was the ultraconservative element because "much as they might regret the royal sanction of a disagreeable modern habit, they could not permit the slightest appearance of disapproval to creep into public view." Added the editor, "The Queen's queenliness is far more important than her smokiness, and cannot be smudged with one tiny streak, not if she smokes straight through a dinner, as so many Americans, particularly women, do." On the other hand, he felt the smokers among English women must have been delighted to read the news, to see "the last trace of reproach" removed from the female smoker. "How can an English mother or teacher reprove the smoking daughter?" wondered the editor. "The most filial child could not be expected to refrain from reminding her elders that the Queen sets the example for the Empire."[6]

An increasing number of women cigarette smokers in Germany, and Europe in general, resulted in a 1929 ruling by the German state railroads requiring that half of the space on every German train was to be designated as smoking compartments. Not long after that, Adolph Hitler and his Nazi regime came to power — and the attitude toward female smokers changed.[7]

Women wearing cosmetics were barred from meetings of the Lower Frankish Nazi women's organizations as of August 1933. Women smokers were expelled from those groups. About a week after that, the police president of Erfurt directed restaurant and café owners to display signs requesting women not to smoke. He also admonished all citizens that they had to cooperate in "stopping this abuse" and declared "when they encounter women smoking they must remind them of their duty as German women and mothers." One month later the city of Erfurt said it was proud of being the first city in Germany to have introduced into places of public entertainment signs reading "The German Woman Does Not Smoke," and gratified at finding imitators. The city councils of Merserberg, Weissensens, and Seitz had all passed resolutions requiring restaurants and cafés to display similar signs. Those resolutions asserted, "according to sound German feeling the mischievous habit of women's smoking is discordant."[8]

Gerhard Wagner, Reich Medical Fuehrer, warned German women in 1937 to refrain from smoking until they were over 50 years of age. He explained that smoking could affect their ability to bear children. Additionally, he warned them to avoid alcohol, except in very small quantities.[9]

As of 1939, minors and women working in German breweries and tobacco factories would no longer be given free beer and free tobacco, respectively. The reason for abandoning the custom was said to be that it "is not in accordance with the most recent interpretations of laws of health and capabilities." Minors and women who worked in tobacco factories, to replace their lost free tobacco, received extra funds for books, vacations, and so forth.[10]

Female students in the Reich were no longer allowed to smoke at the universities they attended as of June 1940. That order was delivered by Dr. Anne Kothenhoff, head of the National Socialist Female Student League, to which all female students had to belong. She said the order was imposed for commonsense reasons because smoking had been scientifically demonstrated to be bad for women. However, a more cogent reason was revealed in the last sentence of her announcement: "Every cigarette that female students do not smoke now saves one for the soldiers on the front." Women students were also admonished to curtail as much as possible their smoking at home.[11]

Under tobacco rationing, as of February 1942, Germans were allowed to have three cigarettes a day, instead of five. However, a tobacco ration was denied to German women.[12]

A war-related tobacco shortage also hit France, beginning in 1941 during the Vichy regime. To be allowed to purchase tobacco in any form, it was necessary to register at cigarette stores in conformity with the newly imposed regulations. Men above the age of 18 alone had the right to register; it meant nonsmoking bachelors suddenly found themselves very popular with the women. After July 16, 1941, only those registered had the right to buy a weekly ration of tobacco — three packs of cigarettes, or three ounces of pipe tobacco, or ten cigars, or four ounces of chewing plug. For some reason the consumption of snuff was not restricted. Each time a registered male made a tobacco purchase he had to fill in a form by writing "I certify that I smoke" or "chew," as the case was.[13]

By late 1944, the Vichy regime had vanished but the tobacco ration system remained in effect. Women were still completely excluded from legally purchasing tobacco; they were agitating to have that changed. Early the following year specific tobacco ration cards were being put into effect in an effort to frustrate women smokers in one of their methods of agitation. As a protest against the discrimination of the tobacco ration system, many women reportedly "corrected" their general ration card, changing their sex by a stroke of the pen, and then used that to register for a tobacco ration.[14]

France's finance minister, Rene Pleven, who presided over the French state tobacco monopoly, courted great unpopularity in July 1945 when he refused tobacco cards to women. In Algiers the French government of Charles de Gaulle had granted equal suffrage to women, who went to the polls in great numbers for the local elections the previous spring. That action by Pleven infuriated many as being a statement that although women could vote, they could not — or should not — smoke. Some thought his decision had something to do with the fact he had "the reputation of being something of a puritan." Pleven told the Consultative Assembly, in explaining the move, "Few women smoke, not more than 10 to 15 per cent. Moreover if they were granted tobacco cards they would simply increase black-market possibilities."[15]

Yet French women scored what was called a victory just two months later when Pleven conceded that they had a right to smoke. Cynical observers noted that not only did women outnumber men in France, but they had been enfranchised and national elections were due in a month. Beginning in December 1945, Pleven announced, women in France would be entitled to the same tobacco ration as men were.[16]

As was the case in America, statistics on the prevalence of women smokers were sparse. A report issued by the British tobacco industry in 1958 said that 41 percent of British women were smokers then, three times the rate found in 1939 (14 percent). As of 1958, 75 percent of British males were reported to be smokers, a number that had not increased at all in the previous 20 years. Men were heavier smokers than women, though. The average male who smoked cigarettes consumed 124 of them per week; the average female went through 71 cigarettes per week.[17]

13

America, 1927–1950

"It yet remains to be seen what a semiparalyzed public will actually do in the face of a menace [smoking by women] that threatens to destroy the finer womanhood of America and permit the realization of that greatest menace to modern civilization, the complete masculinization of womankind."

— F. M. Gregg, 1929

"A large female population, especially in rural areas in the Middle West, has not yet acquired the smoking habit."
— Harry W. Wooten, 1946

Sporadic reports were heard from colleges in this period with a few institutions still engaged in a lonelier and losing battle. However, the issue did not engage the media or the general public the way it had in the first half of the 1920s. By the 1930s, the issue had been settled in the minds of most people; like it or not, women smoked at the institutions of higher learning.

Late in 1929, Dean George W. Stephens at Washington University, St. Louis, Missouri, reiterated a long-standing faculty ruling that smoking by women students was not allowed at Washington University. Speaking before a meeting of the members of campus sororities, the dean declared the rule would be enforced at all university social functions as well. Although the ban against smoking by women on the campus and in sorority houses had reportedly been observed, Stephens said he wanted to "clarify the uncertainty in the minds of some students as to what the university offices are expecting from them."[1]

From Lewisburg, Pennsylvania, came a 1930 report that 44 of the 400 female students at Bucknell University were barred from walking on the campus and having dates for the next six months as a result of their admissions that they smoked in their rooms. That penalty was handed out by a self-governing student organization, the Women's Student Senate, after the 44 had found themselves unable to sign a statement that they had not smoked in their rooms. Although the no-smoking rule was a college order, the investigation was made and the penalty imposed by the self-governing body without the college authorities being involved.[2]

Charles McKenny, president of the Michigan State Normal College (Ypsilanti), told a group of women students in 1931 that no woman known to be a habitual user of cigarettes or who smoked in public places would be allowed to graduate. According to McKenny, the people of Michigan did not want schoolteachers who smoked. Lydia I. Jones, dean of women at the school, added that when a female student was discovered to be even an occasional user of cigarettes, such a fact was noted on her record card and worked against her chances of finding teaching employment after leaving college.[3]

As president of New York City's municipally maintained Hunter College, largest for females in the world with 20,000 students, James M. Kiernan declared, "Smoking hasn't much of a grip on our girls yet. One of our college papers last spring started campaigning for smoking. I remained silent, but this last fall I set aside a smoking room for women." Yet only six to eight were said to use it daily. "By nonresistance it failed to develop into an issue. Most of the girls, therefore, weren't interested."[4]

Through the fall of 1933 smoking by women at Fresno State College had been banned. Females wanting to smoke had to do it in the semi-privacy of their cars or in a booth in a nearby restaurant. Some advocated removing the restrictions on smoking in the Associated Women Students' rooms, so a secret ballot was held; tobacco won by a vote of 310 to 160 (the student body contained about 800 women). Prior to the vote the faculty and the college had agreed to abide by the vote results. Dean Mary Baker said it was better that such a step be taken than to have the women sneak off to smoke in places where they might be seen by children who might later be in their classes when those women became teachers.[5]

A lengthy survey of women-only colleges in 1937 revealed that bans on students smoking were the exception rather than the rule. At Barnard College (New York, Columbia University) smoking was optional in dorm rooms and was allowed in the so-called student section of the campus. Students at Wellesley College (Massachusetts) completed a questionnaire giving their reasons for smoking. In order of importance they were: curiosity, friends did, social considerations, wanted to, pleasure. Smoking had increased among the student body from 53 percent to 70 percent over 1930. Some 82 percent of the smokers inhaled. At St. Mary's College (Notre

Dame, Indiana) Sister Madleva, president of the school, got tired of seeing women sneak down an alley to puff, and she set up and furnished a $2,000 smoking room. Bryn Mawr College (Pennsylvania) permitted smoking in special rooms in dorms, in hall sitting rooms before guests, certain other campus areas, and anywhere off campus except along the main road near Bryn Mawr, and in railroad stations and on trains near Bryn Mawr. More than half of the school's students smoked. At Vassar College (Poughkeepsie, New York) smoking was allowed in dorm smoking rooms, in bedrooms equipped with regulation ashtrays, and in town buildings, with management's consent. Smoking was not permitted in dorm corridors or baths, in public areas of campus, and before academic buildings. About 75 percent of Vassar students reportedly smoked; most inhaled.[6]

Students at Smith College (Northampton, Massachusetts) were allowed to smoke in special house rooms on weekdays and, except during chapel, on Sundays when the head of the house permitted it and when guests were present; on house porches, athletic fields, in the infirmary (with the doctor's permission), in automobiles with guests, and at off-campus food and drink establishments. Sixty-five percent of the Smith students smoked and inhaled. At Sweet Briar College (Lynchburg, Virginia) the rules had been relaxed for several years, although the practice was still prohibited in the dorms because of the fire hazard and "smokers' need for self discipline" (that being a faculty opinion). Smoking was permitted in parlors, recreation halls; it was prohibited in streets, roads and Lynchburg stores, except drugstores and restaurants. Mount Holyoke College (Massachusetts) allowed puffing in dorm smoking rooms, on Pageant Field, in Wilbur Hall, and in town tearooms. More than 50 percent of the Mt. Holyoke female students smoked. At Mills College (Oakland, California) smoking was permitted in the Woodland and Greek Theaters, in the student union building, and in dorm recreation rooms. No smoking was allowed elsewhere on campus or at social functions; when off-campus, the decision as to whether to smoke was left to the dictates of the student's good taste. Officials at Ferry Hall (Chicago) refused to make a statement, but nearby sources reported the school was definitely against smoking, prohibiting it on campus and frowning on it in public. A spokesperson for Trinity College (Washington, D.C.) said that very few girls smoked at the institution. Apparently a no-smoking ban was in place, for the account said that violations, which were infrequent, led to the transgressors being punished by confinement to campus for an indeterminate period.[7]

In the United States in general in this period, more and more women smoked in more and more places. The sales of American tobacco increased fourfold between 1918 and 1928. In 1900 cigarette consumption, as part of the tobacco industry as a whole, was just 2 percent; by 1930 cigarettes accounted for 40 percent of tobacco consumption. Much of that increase achieved by cigarettes was due to the dramatically changing image of the cigarette as more men moved to the cigarette from other forms of tobacco while women took to them, in increasing numbers.[8]

Civilian female employees of the adjutant and inspector's department at the U.S. Marine Corps headquarters in Washington, D.C., were given permission in 1927 to smoke at their desks. Brigadier General Rufus H. Lane, adjutant and inspector of the Marine Corps headquarters, explained that decision by stating that when the issue was raised he was of the opinion that the same rules applied to men with regard to smoking at work should also be applied to women. Some other Marine Corps officials deplored the news coverage resulting from the announcement because they worried people might get the wrong idea that the rule applied to the entire Marine Corps headquarters, and not just one department.[9]

Another 1927 account stated the addition of women to the ranks of U.S. smokers had been largely responsible for the huge increase in cigarette consumption of about 90 percent since 1920. While cigarette output had climbed in 1926 to 550 percent of the 1914 figures, production of cigars, pipe tobacco and chewing tobacco had actually decreased slightly over that period. Net profits available for dividends of four large U.S. tobacco concerns — R.J. Reynolds Tobacco, American Tobacco, Liggett & Myers, and P. Lorillard — rose from $23.2 million in 1914 to $70.5 million in 1926.[10]

Around the same time, another piece detailed the increase in women smoking. Recently, said the reporter, a woman went to the hairdresser in New York City to find all 15 chairs in the place occupied — all 15 women were smoking. While that may have been unusual, it was not unusual to find several women smoking in almost any hairdressing or beauty establishment. Department stores were said to have recognized for some time the fact that many female shoppers wanted to smoke between purchases and had added ashtrays to the furnishing of the women's lounging rooms. "Hotel lobbies belong to women smokers as much as to the men," it was asserted by the reporter. "Theatres have fitted up special smoking rooms for them, but they are not at all confined to these rooms. They can smoke anywhere in the foyers." Women's clubs also allowed the practice, and the women's colleges, with few exceptions, were said to have succumbed when they found a growing number of the students puffing on the sly.[11]

Writing on the prevalence of female smokers in Los Angeles in 1929, columnist Alma Whitaker observed they could be found smoking "boldly" in the foyer of the Figueroa Playhouse between the acts (free cigarettes were supplied) and at most of the other theaters in the area. Additionally, they could be seen at almost any public banquet, although when Princess Gustave of Sweden was in Los Angeles and smoked a cigarette in public at a banquet at the Biltmore Hotel some three years earlier, it reportedly "was news and created quite a little sensation."[12]

Whitaker was an admitted smoker who went so far as to say she had smoked in the past when she rocked her child in its crib. "Whenever, during the course of twenty years of writing, I have referred to women smoking, it has always brought me sheaves of infuriated letters from indignant citizens, who earnestly trusted that I would crusade against this hideous depravity," she recalled. "The one written in this magazine last year brought me dozens ... all deploring that, in mentioning the facts, I had not also furiously, righteously condemned the habit—for women. I was invited to join anti-cigarette leagues galore."[13]

Men were allowed to smoke in the new DAR (Daughters of the American Revolution) headquarters that opened in Washington, D.C., in 1930. In their old building "no smoking" signs were conspicuous and applied to men and women alike. However, men were desired at important musical and dramatic events planned for the new hall and arrangements for their comfort were considered essential. To that end they had been given two smoking rooms in the new building. Women had many "cozy" dress-

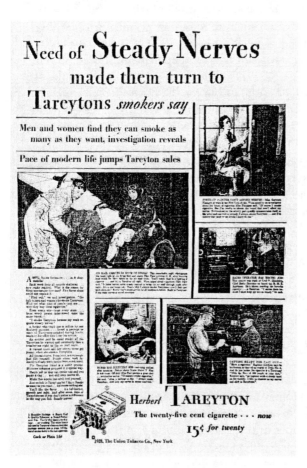

A 1929 appeal to both sexes.

ing rooms, noted an observer, "but none for smoking."[14]

Frances Perkins (she was the U.S. secretary of Labor from 1933 to 1945 under President Franklin D. Roosevelt) declared in a 1930 article that she did not disapprove of women smoking but then went on to mention it created a fire hazard and to score some of them for bad manners. For example, women smoking at the dinner table, through each course, sometimes scattering ashes everywhere but not asking permission to do so, and men were too polite to ask them not to. Perkins believed that department stores had exac-

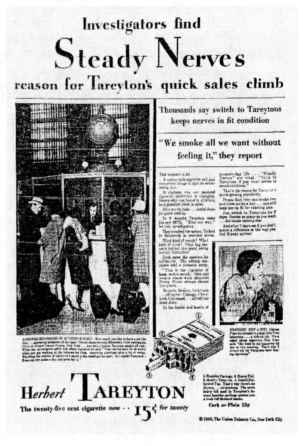

A woman chemist lights up in 1929.

erbated the situation when they put an ashtray beside every chair in the shoe department, and the fitting rooms where they tried on dresses were almost always fitted with smokers' conveniences—increasing the temptation for women carrying cigarettes to smoke. An editor agreed that things were getting worse with the woman smoker being more numerous; "She smokes everywhere — at quick-lunch counters, in dining cars, theatre lobbies, art galleries, street cars and department stores.... It is still unusual for women to smoke as they stroll along the street."[15]

Edmund Brunner of the Manning Publishing Company in Chicago sent out a questionnaire in 1931 to gauge attitudes toward women smokers. Less than 4 percent replied that the average small-town women smoked, although slightly more than half held that smoking was increasing among such women. Some 400 urban ministers and educators, living

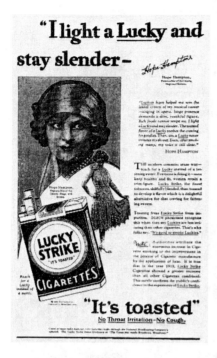 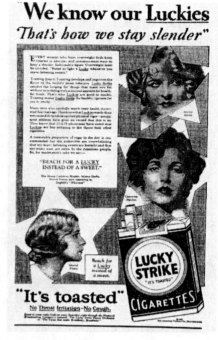

Left: A celebrity endorsement ad, 1929. *Right:* This 1929 ad was another phony one. None of these starlets from the stage show *Whoopee* were smokers of anything.

in cities ranging from 25,000 to 100,000 in population, said that from 20 percent to 60 percent of the women in their communities smoked. Nearly two-thirds of the rural leaders found smoking to be increasing among small-town females, and it was generally held that college women were introducing the cigarette to their rural sisters. Smoking among women, declared Brunner, "is generally regarded as a moral issue in rural communities and is fairly generally regarded as a cause of friction between daughters and mothers."[16]

Advertising trade publication *Printers' Ink* (PI) received a question from one of its readers in early 1932. That reader wanted to know if any data existed on the number of female smokers, how much they smoked, and so forth. PI responded that no surveys had ever been done, so only intelligent guesses could be made. Noting that because women bought and smoked the same brands of cigarettes that men did — that they had never had much to do with the brands made specially for them starting some 20 years earlier and pretty much gone by 1932 — it was almost impossible to determine exactly what percentage of total cigarette consumption was accounted for by females. Back in 1924 PI had published an article by Curtis A. Wessel, managing editor of the trade publication *United States Tobacco Journal*, in which he estimated female consumption then was over three billion cigarettes annually, equal to the total consumption by men 20 years earlier. That estimate applied to 1923 when the total cigarette consumption was over 60 billion, which indicated that women smoked about 5 percent of the total.[17]

PI then commented that in February 1930, Moody's Investors Service published its outlook for the tobacco industry, which included what PI thought was perhaps the first serious effort to arrive at the probable total of cigarettes smoked by women. Said that Moody's report, "We have arrived at the conclusion that women smoked in 1929 not more than 12 per cent of all cigarettes in this country. That is, not more than about 14,000,000,000 cigarettes." In PI's view, cigarette consumption in America had gone through three distinct periods of accelerated growth, with the first being a result of the introduction of blended tobacco (domestic and Turkish) cigarettes in 1912–13. U.S. consumption figures were (in million of cigarettes); 1910, 8,644; 1911, 10,469; 1912, 13,167; 1913, 15,555; 1914, 16,855; almost a doubling of consumption in five years, at a time, said PI, that the majority of women smokers puffed discreetly. The second period of growth came from the effects of World War I (U.S. entry in 1917) 1915, 17,980; 1916, 25,312; 1917, 35,356; 1918, 46,680; and 1919, 53,151. During that period of five years, cigarettes grew dramatically in favor as a man's smoke, at the expense of other forms of tobacco consumption; sending free smokes (bought at home by Americans to ship abroad) to the troops became both a patriotic and fashionable thing to do. Dealing with cigarettes in trenches, at the front, was much easier and more convenient than dealing with tobacco in other forms. Receiving an equality with men — albeit it partial and temporary — in war services and industrial plants helped spur increased smoking by females.[18]

The next period of rapid growth covered the 10 years beginning with 1922 and during which time consumption more than doubled: 1922, 55,780; 1923, 60,862; 1924, 67,884; 1925, 75,011; 1926, 84,941; 1927, 92,976; 1928, 100,584; 1929, 113,985; 1930, 119,941; and 1931, 119,653. The Moody Report noted the gradual concessions made by public opinion with regard to smoking by women, particularly in public places. And although that change took place earlier in Europe than here, the Moody study said that it was not before 1923 and 1924 that widespread smoking among women in the United States began. PI, in its conclusion to the reader's query as to statistics, stated that in view of what had happened since the 1929 Moody estimate (more increases among women) women's consumption must have been higher than 12 percent, putting its own estimate at females having consumed at least 14 percent of all cigarettes in 1931, but that female smokers consumed considerably less cigarettes per day than did the male puffers. "Therefore, it would not be safe to assume that 14 percent of cigarette smokers are women; the actual percentage is likely to be considerably higher."[19]

A *Fortune* magazine survey in 1935 found that 52.5 percent of men and 18.1 percent of women reported themselves to be cigarette smokers; those figures varied with the respondent's age and place of residence. Among women under 40 years of age, 26.2 percent smoked; 9.3 percent of women over 40 indulged. Women's smoking was more common in cities with populations between 100,000 and 1 million (40.2 percent) and least common in rural areas (8.6 percent).[20]

An inspector with the federal government Internal Revenue Service, based in Washington, D.C., spotted a female worker in the St. Louis office smoking while on duty and complained there to collector Thomas J. Sheehan. After an inquiry, it was revealed that although the rules prohibited men employees from smoking on duty, no rule existed relating to women, who then promptly cited the 19th Amendment to the Constitution (women's suffrage) in their own defense. A compromise was reached when Sheehan outfitted a smoking room for the women.[21]

In response to a threatened war-related cigarette shortage near the end of 1944, U.S. Representative Clare Booth Luce of Connecticut urged American women to give up one cigarette daily to help alleviate any warfront smoking shortage, which she saw in evidence during a congressional party's tour — Luce made her plea from Paris. "I myself have cut out smoking in the morning," she added.[22]

When the American Institute of Public Opinion conducted a national survey of smoking habits in 1944, it found that 52 percent of the adult civilian population smoked tobacco, mostly cigarettes. Men in the armed forces were excluded from the survey. Nearly two-thirds of all adult women interviewed in the survey did not smoke at all. Among civilian men, the number who had never taken up the habit, or had sworn off, was only about one in four. Farm areas and small towns had the lowest proportion of smokers per 1,000 population, whereas large cities had the highest level. A higher proportion of white-collar workers smoked cigarettes than any other single occupational group. Among civilian adults aged 20 to 26, 55 percent smoked cigarettes, as compared with only 25 percent among people aged 50 and over.[23]

Making some postwar pronouncements in 1946, Harry W. Wooten, tobacco consultant and sales analyst, predicted American cigarette manufacturers would concentrate sales efforts in the next two years "on a virtually untapped market among women in the Middle West." While smoking among women in the East and on the Pacific Coast "is quite prevalent," said Wooten, "a large female population, especially in rural areas in the Middle West, has not yet acquired the smoking habit." Consumption of cigarettes in the U.S. domestic market was 332 billion, Wooten reported. He hoped, if women could be recruited, to see that number reach 400 billion yearly. At its peak the U.S. armed forces market absorbed 11.6 billion cigarettes monthly.[24]

Wooten's remarks caused the *Christian Science Monitor* to editorialize, "Time was, not so many years ago, when tobacco advertisers had to tread softly on women's natural distaste for a habit which was considered far from dainty or wholesome." He continued that the large-scale promotion Wooten suggested would be directed at Midwestern women "will seek to add to tobacco profits while it serves to detract yet further from feminine charm and freshness. But at least the proposed victims have been warned."[25]

Pollster George Gallup commented in 1946: "Take the matter of smoking. It is generally accepted today that women have a right to smoke." When the Gallup poll put the issue of women teachers and smoking before public opinion, the women were victorious. The American Institute of Public Opinion asked respondents: "The school boards in many communities do not allow women teachers to smoke. Do you think this rule should be changed to allow women teachers to smoke while outside the classroom?" Sixty-two percent said yes, 32 percent said no, 6 percent were undecided. Among no group and in no part of the country, except the 13 states comprising the South, did more people vote to keep teachers from smoking than voted in favor of allowing them to smoke.[26]

Another Gallup poll conducted by the American Institute of Public Opinion in 1949 found that cigarette smoking among the young was almost twice as great as among the elderly. Respondents across America were asked, "Do you happen to smoke cigarettes now?" Nationally the yes response was 44 percent; men, 54 percent; women, 33 percent; 21–29 year olds, 51 percent; 30–49 year olds, 52 percent; 50 and over, 28 percent. Each cigarette smoker was asked how many he or she smoked per day; the average of all replies was 17 cigarettes. According to the U.S. Department of Agriculture, American consumption of cigarettes in 1949 was 358 billion. All respondents in the poll were asked, "Do you think cigarette smoking is harmful or not?" Among cigarette smokers, 52 percent said it was harmful, 45 percent said not harmful, 3 percent had no opinion. For non-cigarette smokers the numbers were, respectively, 66 percent, 24 percent, and 10 percent.[27]

A large survey by the U.S. Bureau of the Census for the National Cancer Institute in 1955 revealed that some 38 million Americans smoked cigarettes regularly, including 13 million women. About 50 percent of U.S. men and 25 percent of women smoked cigarettes daily. Another estimate was that about 1 million men and 500,000 women stopped cigarette smoking entirely since the fall of 1953 due to "scary" reports linking lung cancer to cigarette smoking and linking the habit with heart disease and heart deaths.[28]

A report in 1960 said that smoking in America had reached a record level, with the nation having 58 million smokers, 58 percent of all men and 36 percent of all women over age 15. In 1959 Americans consumed a record 462.7 billion cigarettes, up 4.5 percent from a record-setting pace in 1958.[29]

Public Places

When 15 English women, all department buyers for Harrods of London, the famous department store, arrived in Chicago on a buying trip in the summer of 1927, they lodged at the Congress Hotel. One day those women were smoking in the lobby, but the manager came over to advise them it was against the rules. They were told that smoking rooms were available for women and that they were also permitted to smoke in the hotel's cafés. However, they insisted on smoking in the lobby along with all the men who were allowed to puff away there and were doing so. "In England it is etiquette for women to smoke anywhere. We will smoke in the lobby or go to another hotel," said one of the women. "Evidently Americans wish their women to smoke in private but not in public," complained another member of the group, Gertrude Heaton. "Never before have we run into anything like this. You would think we had bad reputations— to be stopped like this from smoking in the lobby." Later on the party toured the big Chicago department stores and were not impressed with the amount of time permitted the employees for rest breaks. In Harrods, they said, the clerks were given coffee and opportunity to smoke and relax at 10:30 in the morning and again in the afternoon at 4:00, a half hour for tea and cigarettes.[30]

When Alonzo B. See, Brooklyn elevator manufacturer, visited the Lake Placid Club in New York City in 1927, he read on the menu this sentence: "Smoking by women not allowed either in the building or on club grounds." Later he wrote to the president of that club to commend him on the rule. "I never question women's right to smoke. It is not a question of right — it goes beyond that," he stated. "It is a question of what is best for the women. Women began smoking because they think it looks smart. But it soon becomes with them a disease." See also mentioned a woman at a New York dinner he attended who had smoked "incessantly" through the dinner and the following speeches with the result "she was torpid during the entire time of the dinner and speeches and looked as she sagged back in her chair like

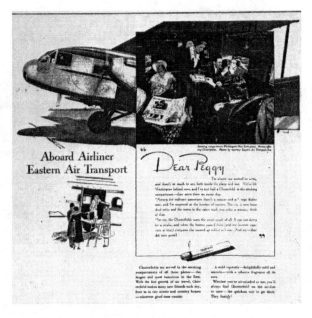

Passengers smoking on a plane in a 1931 ad. The flight attendant passed out free smokes.

the pictures we have seen of Chinamen as they lay in the drowsy state smoking the opium in their pipes."[31]

The popularity of cigarette smoking among women caused several department stores in the Southern United States to sell cigarettes by vending machines in 1928 — those machines, fairly new on the scene, were just becoming a big fad. Consolidated Automatic Merchandising Corporation announced it had signed contracts with Thalhimer Brothers (Richmond, Virginia) and D. H. Holmes Company (New Orleans), for the installation of vending machines in their stores.[32]

An appeal was made in December 1936 by New York City fire commissioner John J. McElligott to the heads of all the large department stores in the city to enlist their stores in a "no-smoking" campaign to minimize as far as possible the ever-present danger of fire. He said he received letters of complaint almost daily from shoppers worried about the situation in the stores. McElligott's letter to each store read, in part, "While I appreciate that there is no ordinance prohibiting smoking in department stores of this kind and while I personally am not advocating such an ordinance, I am hoping that you will adopt a policy preventing smoking by shoppers." When he spoke to reporters, McElligott told them something that was absent from the letters. He said the danger lay not with men "who know

A 1929 ad by various parts of the food industry, outraged by the Lucky Strike campaign for people to smoke rather than eat. It demanded to have such campaigns removed from radio. Eventually the FTC did bar Lucky Strike from making such unfounded claims as saying that smoking could make you thin.

how to smoke," but with women "who don't know how to smoke. I personally never have seen one who did and enjoyed it. Ladies hold a cigarette in one hand and handle flimsy stuff with the other."[33]

A 30-year ban on smoking at the State Reformatory for Women in Bedford, New York, was lifted in 1933 by Dr. P. E. Battey, superintendent

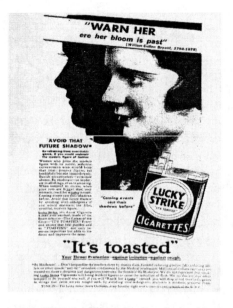

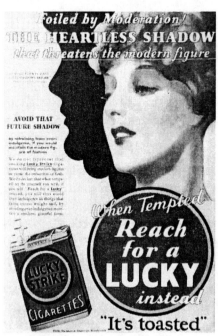

Two 1930 ads still on the slim theme. Note the double chins on the shadows but not on the faces — the shape of things to come.

of the facility. He reasoned that because the outside world permitted smoking by women, there was therefore little reason for continuing the prohibition in the reformatory. Female detainees whose deportment remained satisfactory were permitted to smoke in specially designated parts of the institutional buildings from that time onward. In the female homes for correction, the prisoners were allowed to smoke, remarked Battey. And he thought that was another reason why the ban should be lifted.[34]

Street smoking by women could still cause problems for them right into the 1930s, although that last taboo was also disappearing and was gone before this period ended. Illustrating that taboo and the lengths some women went to avoid it was a summer 1927 account that declared a few years earlier an enterprising taxi driver did a thriving business in the Wall Street district of New York during the noon hour by driving around women who wanted to smoke a cigarette or two before returning to their offices. None of the women rode any considerable distance, but the taxi driver had a continual run of passengers. According to the story, the taxi was about the only place these women could smoke with any sense of freedom. "In the restaurants they would have felt conspicuous. In the offices it was quite out of the question. An unwritten law said that women must not smoke in business houses." Comparing that situation with the one in the year he was writing, 1927, the reporter observed, "Today there is hardly any place except the street where women cannot smoke with equanimity."[35]

Edward Bernays, a seminal figure in American advertising and public relations in the 20th century, the father of the modern form of that industry in many eyes, related a story about women and street smoking in his autobiography. According to Bernays, "In 1929 it was acceptable for women to smoke at home, but a woman seen smoking in public was labeled a hussy or worse." George Washington Hill, president of American Tobacco— Lucky Strike was the brand —called him in as a public relations counsel to do something about the situation because Hill thought he could increase his market greatly if women would smoke on the street. Bernays called in Dr. A. A. Brill, the psychoanalyst, who explained that some women smoked because they regarded cigarettes as symbols of freedom or "torches of freedom." So Bernays decided on a parade of women lighting torches of freedom — smoking cigarettes— and the 1929 Easter Sunday Parade on Fifth Avenue in New York City seemed a natural place to launch it. In his version 10 debutantes marched from 48th Street to 54th Street "as a protest against women's inequality and caused a national stir. Front-page stories in newspapers reported the freedom march in words and pictures. For weeks after the event editorials praised or condemned the young women who had paraded against the smoking taboo." Bernays continued, "The demonstration became almost a

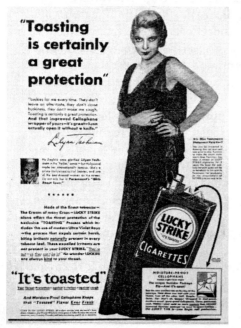

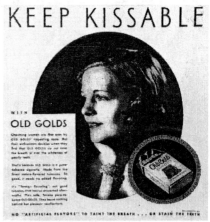

Left: A 1931 endorsement ad. *Above:* How to stay kissable in 1931.

national issue…. Women's clubs throughout the country expressed grief that women would smoke in public; papers in Boston, Detroit, Wheeling, West Virginia, and San Francisco reported women smoking on the streets as a result of the New York parade."[36]

To this day, some accounts use the Bernays story as evidence he was an important figure in getting more women to smoke, and so on. The problem was that nothing Bernays wrote about the reaction to the parade seemed to have happened, although the event itself did happen. A very long article about that Easter Parade appeared in the *New York Times* on April 1, 1929. Running to perhaps 2,000 words, it discussed such things as what types of sermons had been delivered in area churches, by whom, activities in other nearby areas, and, of course, the timeless staple of such articles— long descriptions of what people were wearing, ordinary folk for the most part. Easter Parades of the era were occasions for ordinary people to dress up in their finest clothes, attend church, and then "parade" around a bit, as opposed to the usual type of parade where most people passively observed. Buried two-thirds of the way through that story was a very brief mention of the Bernays publicity effort; "About a dozen young women strolled back and forth between St. Thomas's and St. Patrick's while the parade was at its peak, ostentatiously smoking cigarettes. Two were asked which brand they favored, and they named it. One of the group explained the cigarettes were 'torches of freedom' lighting the way to the day when women would smoke on the street as casually as men."[37]

Despite Bernays's claim that the stunt generated much publicity, nothing else could be found. No national magazine (of those indexed by the *Reader's Guide* periodical index) carried so much as a mention of the incident. The *New York Times* mention was limited to the quote above; it said no more then or later on the subject. Also, there was not a single word about the incident to be found in the following newspapers: the *Christian Science Monitor,* the *Wall Street Journal,* the *Washington Post,* or the *Los Angeles Times.* No publicity was generated by the stunt because the issue of females smoking had been settled — in their favor — with a dwindling number of individual objectors. Street smoking had not fully fallen, but the nonreaction to Bernays's stunt indicated it was a rapidly disintegrating taboo.

New York magistrate George B. Deluca fined a man $25 in 1931 for knocking a cigarette from a woman's mouth as she puffed away in the street on Park Avenue in New York City. Pearl Barton yelled for a policeman after Michael Kelleher had knocked away her cigarette. Revealed in court, also, was that Kelleher stamped on Barton's feet and "spoiled" her hat and dress while she was hanging on to him awaiting the arrival of the law. In the view of the headline writer of the account reporting the Barton incident Magistrate Deluca's finding indicated, "Smoking of women on streets is upheld."[38]

Residents of the small community of Northumberland in Pennsylvania were reported to have been "astonished" in 1934 when they saw a woman strolling down the street smoking a pipe. The chief of police was summoned. However, he informed the residents that nothing could be done, as there was no law in that jurisdiction to prevent women from smoking.[39]

An editorial in the *New York Times* of June 28, 1949, commented on the "vast number" of women to be seen smoking on the streets of New York City, "and drawing no particular comment." He felt there were just as many women smoking on the streets as men, maybe more. It had not always been that way, he added.[40]

Medical Opinion

Medical advice offered in this period continued to present the habit almost completely in a negative light, with an emphasis on the effects of the practice on babies. Weirdness in such opinion was not absent. One of the more outrageous opinions came from Dr. Charles L. Barber, of Lansing, Michigan, at the annual convention of the American Association for Medico-Physical Research in Chicago in 1927. He told attendees that 60 percent of all babies born to cigarette-smoking mothers died before they reached the age of two, due primarily to nicotine poisoning. "A baby born of a cigarette-smoking mother is sick," he declared. "It is poisoned and may die within two weeks of birth. The postmortem shows degeneration of the liver, heart and other organs. Sixty per cent of all babies born of cigarette-smoking mothers will die before they are 2 years old."[41]

Doctors criticizing other doctors

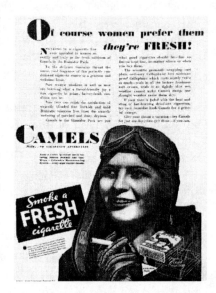

1931. When women models were used to endorse cigarettes they were usually depicted as physically active in some way.

were rare but Barber's comments provoked a large number of New York specialists who took "sharp issue" with his assertions. Dr. Oscar M. Schloss dismissed the claim as "absurd." Infant mortality in New York then was about 5 in 1,000. More diplomatic was Dr. Charles Hendee Smith, who said of the claim, "It is certainly exaggerated." He added that although he had no definite statistics concerning the offspring of smoking and nonsmoking mothers, his experience had been that a good many healthy and husky babies were born of mothers who smoked cigarettes. On the other hand, he added that he had seen many fragile and weak babies born of mothers who had never used tobacco.[42]

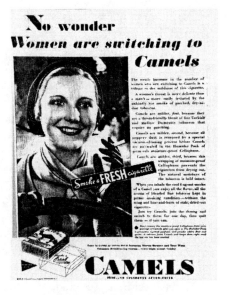

1931. This ad argued that a woman's throat was different from a man's.

Even an official publication of the American Medical Association (*Hygeia*, for the layperson) felt compelled to comment. With respect to Barber's organization, *Hygeia* declared, "This is an organization of nondescript practitioners of healing, representing the outgrowth of a moribund, if not defunct, society developed by the late but not greatly lamented Albert Abrams, founder of the so-called electronic medicine." Once upon a time, said the article, newspapers devoted columns to the vagarious notions uttered at such conventions, but editors had since become better informed and usually then ignored such pronouncements. As far as Barber's 60 percent claim went, asserted *Hygeia*, "This announcement is supported by evidence like that regularly used to convince the credulous that the moon is made of green, and not limburger, cheese. As a scientific statement, it partakes of the odor popularly credited to the second mentioned form of fromage." Nevertheless, rued the magazine,

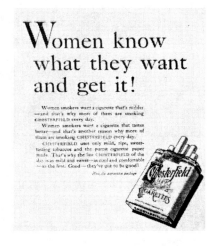

1931 plain talk.

the claim by Barber was broadcast throughout the nation by several press services and selected by a few editors "who should have known better." No purpose could be served by the item except possibly "to stimulate still further anticigarette fanatics."[43]

Reporting in 1935 on experiments they had conducted at Antioch College, Drs. Lester W. Sontag and Robert F. Wallace declared that when a mother smoked heavily before the birth of her child, some of the substance in tobacco smoke that made the heart beat faster was transmitted to the blood of her unborn child and also made its heart beat faster. In their scientific report the physicians made no statement concerning the harmful effects of maternal smoking on the unborn child. But, they told reporters, taking into consideration the work of other scientists on the effects of nicotine in the milk of smoking mothers, they considered it "not improbable" that maternal smoking before the birth of the child may have permanently harmful effects on the offspring.[44]

At the 1942 meeting of the American Medical Association, Dr. H. Harris Perlman of Philadelphia reported a study on the effect of cigarette smoking on the milk and infants of nursing mothers. Perlman said the study showed that nicotine was excreted in the milk and urine of all the mothers who smoked cigarettes and that there was a definite correlation between the quantity of nicotine excreted and the number of cigarettes smoked. The supply of milk from the mothers was little, if at all, affected by smoking cigarettes. He added that the infants were apparently unaffected by the quantity of nicotine they obtained through the milk.[45]

William Brady, a medical doctor who wrote a newspaper advice column in the mid–1940s and a smoker himself, offered the thought that women were more likely to indulge to excess in cigarette smoking than were men. Brady did mention the dangers of "secondhand" smoke indoors to

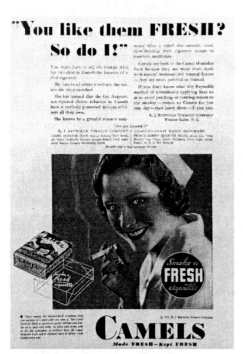

A 1932 ad featured a model that was not a nurse but designed to convince the reader, by indirection, that she was.

the elderly, the infirm, young children, and so on. He added that some physicians appeared to regard smoking as not particularly harmful to the expectant or nursing mother or her baby, whereas others regarded it as harmful. "If you ask me, I say the less smoking you or anyone does in the house or room with the baby the better for the health of all concern," he concluded.[46]

Adverse effects on beauty were noted again. Dr. Herbert Schlink, surgeon of the Royal Prince Albert Hospital in Australia, said in a 1928 interview in Boston that American women were seriously injuring their beauty and health by excessive cigarette smoking. Women who

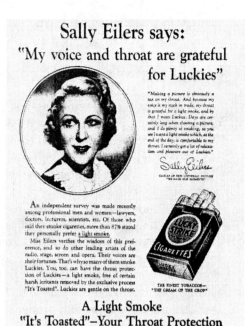

More preposterous claims, 1937.

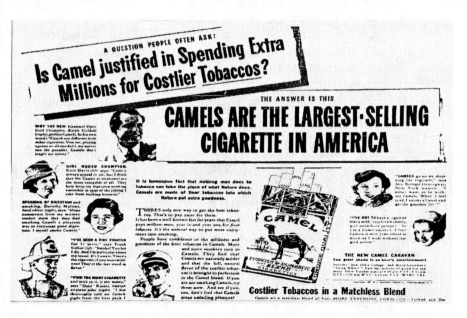

1937. Featured in this ad were a "girl" rodeo champion and a "girl" parachute jumper.

smoked incessantly, he stated, were becoming neurotic and typical "nerve" subjects for hospitals and specialists, not only in the United States, but also throughout the world.[47]

Delegates to the cosmeticians' convention in Chicago in 1931 were told by Mrs. M. B. McGavran, president of the American Association of Cosmeticians, that cigarette smoking was giving American women a "bloodhound facial drop." She explained, "Women smokers' faces are growing sharper. Lips are becoming pallid, corners of the mouth sag, lips commence to protrude and develop twitching habits and the eyes acquire a blank stare."[48]

Journalist Allan Benson remarked in 1929 on the dramatic increase in the number of female smokers and that it was a common sight then, at least in the business offices of New York, to see young girls sitting at their desks smoking. He asked some medical doctors about the habit. Dr. R. A. Bartholomew, associate professor at Emory University School of Medicine told him, "I feel there is a decided tendency for overindulgence in smoking among women. This is due to the fact that they have more leisure time." Bartholomew related it was known that nicotine increased blood pressure, over stimulated heart action, produced catarrhal conditions in the respiratory passages, reduced the appetite "and furthermore the nervous effects are apt to be more marked on account of the more delicate nervous system of the average woman. So far as I know, there is no experimental work on which to base an opinion as to the harmful effects on the unborn child, but my feeling is that it may be definitely harmful."[49]

Dr. Bernard Fantus, associate professor at Chicago's Rush Medical College told Benson, "One who is slightly old-fashioned can hardly associate with his idea of dainty womanhood the coated tongue, offensive breath, the hawking and spitting resulting from inflammation of the mouth and throat that habitual excessive smoking is bound to produce." Said Dr. Floyd W. Rice of Des Moines, Iowa, "As to the physical effect on the smoking woman, the physician needs but to observe her — nervous, underweight, sallow-complexioned, with a poor appetite, hacking cough, dark circles under the eyes, husky-voiced, suffering from sleeplessness, and irritable." He added that when he discovered the habit in one of his patients and induced her to quit, she became "plump, bright-eyed, healthy complexioned, clear-voiced, happy and contented. The improvement was miraculous." Benson concluded by expressing a worry that more females would fall victim to cigarette advertising than would males because "they have certain temperamental qualities that make them particularly susceptible to shrewd advertising appeal."[50]

Lydia Lane also had a newspaper advice column. In a 1935 column she presented a "famous doctor's" rules for smoking. They were: don't smoke until past the teen years; don't smoke more than eight cigarettes a day; do not inhale; use a cigarette holder, as it helps filter out nicotine; stop smoking for a month at least once a year; and never smoke during meals. Lane concluded that while much had been said on the subject, "no definite and serious harm has ever been proven to cigarette smoking in moderation. So remember the six rules and you need not worry about your heart, your complexion or your digestion."[51]

An article in *Hygeia* in 1948 said that coronary thrombosis had increased sharply among women and that "smoking may have something to do" with it. Men once developed that form of heart disease from 50 to 60 times as frequently as women, but by the late 1940s one woman had the condition for every three men.[52]

Dr. Joseph Colt Bloodgood, noted cancer specialist of the Johns Hopkins University Hospital faculty, was asked in 1928 about statements by surgeons made before the Association of Osteopathic Physicians at Tampa that cancer of the lips of women who smoked was presenting a serious problem. Bloodgood declared, "Women who smoke in moderation need not be alarmed. It is only when an irritation develops on the lip that they should cease smoking."[53]

Then, in the early 1950s, the situation got worse as more medical reports linked smoking to serious health problems. Much more serious attention was devoted to those reports. It was not apparent in the very early 1950s, but smoking had started a reverse journey. Cigarette smoking had moved from pariah status to bosom companion to equality among the sexes from about 1880 to 1950. Now it was starting the return trip; it was heading back to pariah status. Typical of those early 1950s medical warnings was one from Dr. Edgar Mayer, clinical professor of medicine at New York University Postgraduate Medical Center. He declared, "The evidence is strongly supportive that smoking does" play an important part in causing lung cancers. Lung cancer cases had doubled in the 20 years from 1930 to 1950, from 15,000 to 30,000 cases, he observed. And the fact that six times as many men as women had lung cancer could be indicative because women had been smoking excessively only for about 10 or 15 years. In his view consuming one or two packs a day was excessive smoking. Mayer smoked half a pack a day himself.[54]

Advertising

For the first time, beginning roughly in 1927, advertising of tobacco that directly and indirectly targeted women became an issue. It became an

Jane Wyatt says:

"Luckies are a light smoke my throat approves
and my taste prefers"

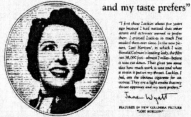

An independent survey was made recently among professional men and women—lawyers, doctors, lecturers, scientists, etc. Of those who said they smoke cigarettes, more than 87% stated they personally prefer a light smoke.

Miss Wyatt verifies the wisdom of this preference, and so do other leading artists of the radio, stage, screen and opera. Their voices are their fortunes. That's why so many of them smoke Luckies. You, too, can have the throat protection of Luckies—a light smoke, free of certain harsh irritants removed by the exclusive process "It's Toasted". Luckies are gentle on the throat.

THE FINEST TOBACCO—
"THE CREAM OF THE CROP"

A Light Smoke
"It's Toasted"–Your Throat Protection
AGAINST IRRITATION–AGAINST COUGH

Barbara Stanwyck says:

"Luckies make a hit with
my throat"

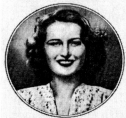

An independent survey was made recently among professional men and women—lawyers, doctors, lecturers, scientists, etc. Of those who said they smoke cigarettes, more than 87% stated they personally prefer a light smoke.

Miss Stanwyck verifies the wisdom of this preference, and so do other leading artists of the radio, stage, screen and opera. Their voices are their fortunes. That's why so many of them smoke Luckies. You, too, can have the throat protection of Luckies—a light smoke, free of certain harsh irritants removed by the exclusive process "It's Toasted". Luckies are gentle on the throat.

THE FINEST TOBACCO—
"THE CREAM OF THE CROP"

A Light Smoke
"It's Toasted"–Your Throat Protection
AGAINST IRRITATION–AGAINST COUGH

Carole Lombard says:

"Advised by my singing coach,
I changed to Luckies"

An independent survey was made recently among professional men and women—lawyers, doctors, lecturers, scientists, etc. Of those who said they smoke cigarettes, more than 87% stated they personally prefer a light smoke.

Miss Lombard verifies the wisdom of this preference, and so do other leading artists of the radio, stage, screen and opera. Their voices are their fortunes. That's why so many of them smoke Luckies. You, too, can have the throat protection of Luckies—a light smoke, free of certain harsh irritants removed by the exclusive process "It's Toasted". Luckies are gentle on the throat.

THE FINEST TOBACCO—
"THE CREAM OF THE CROP"

A Light Smoke
"It's Toasted"–Your Throat Protection
AGAINST IRRITATION–AGAINST COUGH

Elisabeth Rethberg
finds voice and throat safe with Luckies

*Famous Metropolitan
Opera Soprano writes:*

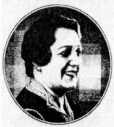

An independent survey was made recently among professional men and women—lawyers, doctors, lecturers, scientists, etc. Of those who said they smoke cigarettes, more than 87% stated they personally prefer a light smoke.

Miss Rethberg verifies the wisdom of this preference, and so do other leading artists of the radio, stage, screen and opera. Their voices are their fortunes. That's why so many of them smoke Luckies. You, too, can have the throat protection of Luckies—a light smoke, free of certain harsh irritants removed by the exclusive process "It's Toasted". Luckies are gentle on the throat.

THE FINEST TOBACCO—
"THE CREAM OF THE CROP"

A Light Smoke
"It's Toasted"–Your Throat Protection
AGAINST IRRITATION–AGAINST COUGH

1937 endorsements by Jane Wyatt, Barbara Stanwyck, Carole Lombard, and Elizabeth Rethberg.

issue then because prior to that time it had been close to nonexistent. In a related move, the motion picture industry came under attack for what was seen to be an increasing proportion of female screen characters depicted as being cigarette smokers and a shift in the types of characters who smoked, away from the bad girl and toward the good girl. Such depictions were assailed and criticized for being indirect advertising — while no particular brand was touted or identified, such depictions represented little more than advertisements for the general practice of cigarette smoking.

Ralph S. Bauer, described as Lynn, Massachusetts's "moral crusader" mayor, announced in October 1929 that he was banning the exhibition in local cinemas of motion pictures showing women or girls smoking cigarettes. Bauer had, around the same time, caused to be removed from his city a billboard that showed a sailor and a young woman consuming the weed. Among his other accomplishments was to put a ban on bare female knees and to have issued an edict against "automobile sheiks and philandering husbands."[55]

At a 1930 convention of the Los Angeles District Federation of Women's Clubs (groups affiliated with that body had a total membership of over 400,000 members) delegates passed a resolution "banning" films that showed women smoking and those showing the serving and drinking of intoxicating liquors. Presumably, they were banned only in the sense the resolution urged affiliated women not to attend the screening of such movies.[56]

In Lincoln, Nebraska, in early 1933, Representative A. A. Heater introduced a bill that, if passed, would have barred any movie showing women smoking cigarettes from being exhibited in Nebraska. Although the proposal failed to pass, it came very close with the final vote result being a tie. A commentator speculated a bill such as Heater's could have been inspired by some such scene as the one in *Mata Hari* where Ramon Novarro and Greta Garbo "seductively conveyed the idea of seduction by the gleam of their lighted cigarettes in a darkened room."[57]

Motion pictures were declared by Maude M. Aldrich, in a 1938 report to the WCTU convention, to be "probably the most powerful medium in putting the cigarette between the lips of American women." Her report urged the convention to support the "proper regulation" of motion pictures."[58]

In the 1930s and 1940s smoking was supported and publicized by many film stars such as Greta Garbo, Bette Davis, and Katherine Hepburn, to mention only a few, and the likes of Rudolph Valentino, Gary Cooper, Humphrey Bogart, Fred Astaire, J. Edgar Hoover, Franklin Delano Roosevelt and Eleanor Roosevelt. It was in the 1930s that it was documented

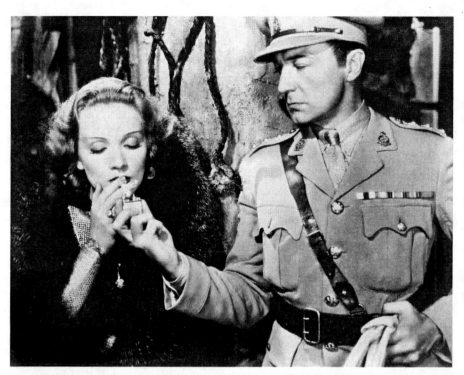

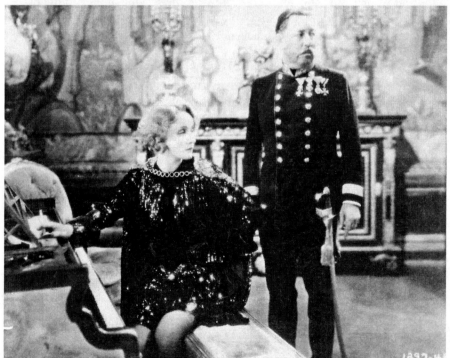

that heroes and heroines in films were much more likely to smoke than were the villains. An analysis of 40 films in the mid–1930s found that 65 percent of the heroes in those movies smoked, compared to 22.5 percent of the villains, while 30 percent of the heroines indulged, against only 2.5 percent of the bad girls. What that suggested was that given the conservative nature of the motion picture industry (it strived to please all and to reflect trends, not set them), cigarette smoking by the 1930s had attained a high level of acceptability among the general public.[59]

Many observers commented on the fact that there was very little advertising of tobacco directed to women before 1927. Writing in 1929, journalist Eunice Fuller Barnard said "So strong, however, remained the prejudice against women smoking in some sections of the country that it was not until 1927 that the large cigarette manufacturers dared to openly direct their advertising to their biggest class of new prospects—the feminine half of the community."[60]

Allan M. Brandt argued that before the late 1920s, social conventions had restricted advertisers from explicitly hyping the cigarette to women. But by the last years of the 1920s those hesitations, due to convention and social mores, among the tobacco advertisers had yielded to a widespread recognition that the increased number of women already smoking presented a potential vast new market for their brand; a potential that was large enough to cause them to start to defy convention.[61]

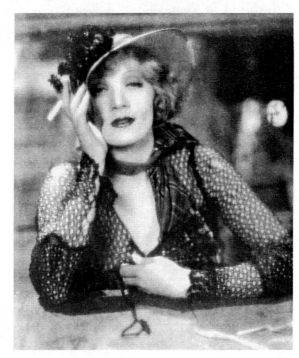

The trade publication *Advertising & Selling* featured an article in a 1926 issue titled "Why cigarette makers don't advertise to women." In that article L. Bonner stated: "The cigarette

Opposite top: Marlene Dietrich and Clive Brook in *Shanghai Express*, 1932. *Opposite bottom:* Marlene Dietrich and Victor McLaglen in *Dishonored*, 1931. *Right:* Marlene Dietrich in *Blond Venus*, 1932.

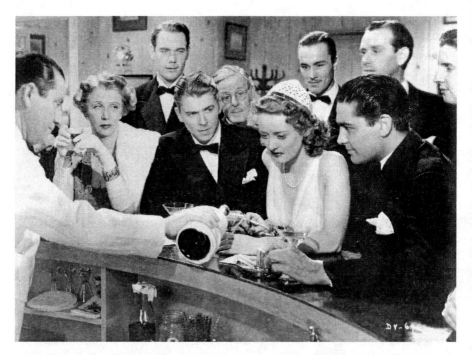

Dark Victory, 1939; Bette Davis right center with cigarette, Ronald Reagan center.

people are frankly afraid of stirring up the reformers and bringing down upon themselves a lot of nuisance legislation." That article predicted that public opinion would soon be on the side of the tobacco industry, and that within a year or two direct advertising appeals to women would be appearing on billboards and in magazines and newspapers. It was a prediction that turned out to be accurate.[62]

A few ads did target females before 1927. One of the first such advertisements was for the Helmar brand of cigarettes in 1919 (manufactured by the Lorillard company). That ad featured the drawing of a woman (with obvious Caucasian features) dressed in Oriental garb and with a cigarette held between her lips. In 1921 a hosiery advertisement that showed a woman displaying the merchandise, and also smoking a cigarette, was said to have "aroused much criticism on Main Street." Even when it was obvious that there were significant numbers of women smoking, declared *Printers' Ink*, "advertisers egged the habit along with the greatest delicacy." An example of that subtlety was to be found in a 1926 Chesterfield ad that showed a couple in a romantic setting: The man was depicted smoking while the woman in a sensuous pose requested of the man, "Blow some my way." By that latter year it was not uncommon to find women depicted in tobacco ads but only as background. They never interacted directly or indirectly with the cigarette (as they did in the Chesterfield ad), functioned only to complete a family grouping, and so on. Marlboro cigarettes, around this time, had as one of their slogans, "Mild as May," which many took as being an indirect appeal to women puffers and potential smokers.[63]

It was likely true that cigarette makers refrained form targeting women with their ads until around 1927 because of a fear of arousing further backlash and criticism from society. It was then only a decade since the cigarette had undergone its final rehabilitation and started down the road to social acceptability. Many states had enacted legislation against the sale of cigarettes to adults (virtually all had done so with respect to sales to minors). Even though bans of sales to adults were rarely ever enforced they were a nuisance and, as long as they remained on state statute books, posed a potential danger to the makers. With the repeal of the last of those laws—Kansas in 1927—the cigarette makers understood the battle was over, symbolically and in reality. No such laws would be enacted again. Cigarette manufacturers understood the new freedom and license that had been won unofficially; they could increase advertising in general and target new groups previously untargeted—such as women. The idea of women smoking had always provoked more criticism and outrage than did the concept of men smoking. Any cigarette advertiser who had targeted women with its ads any time much before 1927 would have run a risk of stirring up a huge public backlash, and no one knew where that might lead. The reward was not worth the risk. But by 1927 the anticigarette lobby had been reduced to a group of weak individuals and groups, increasingly seen as pests and eccentrics. Also, by 1927, there were a lot more female smokers. The debate had carried on in colleges for years and was over by then; most colleges permitted females to smoke somewhere on the campuses, and many of them smoked. By 1927 the rewards of targeting women with ads far outweighed the risks. A check of Literary Digest for January through March for the odd years 1921 through 1929 revealed no tobacco ads that directly or indirectly targeted women. Also checked was American Magazine for January through June, for the odd years from 1915 onward. The first ad therein that pitched cigarettes directly to women appeared in February 1929. More appeared later that year and in every year thereafter.

A reporter commented in August 1927 that the rivalry among cigarette makers had begun to intensify and was apparent in the widened scope of their advertising. "Guardedly and cautiously, the advertising message is beginning to reach out to the woman smoker, who now furnishes a large source of demand, and a wide potential market for the future."[64]

Advertising & Selling had a piece in January 1927 in which O. Williamson discussed with obvious disdain "the firm-rooted belief in the reactionary mind that women — decent, respectable women — do not smoke." Williamson asserted, "There can be but little doubt of the way the wind is beginning to blow, and with such a market awaiting the manufacturer we may expect almost any day to see him right after it." By early 1927 ads making direct appeals to women began to appear in magazines and newspapers. Assisting in that was the decision of the magazine *Pictorial Review* (like other mass circulation women's magazines of the day, it had refused tobacco advertising) to accept such material beginning with the May 1927 issue. Various approaches were used to encourage women to buy their product; testimonials from famous women — from opera stars to actresses, from sports figures to socialites — attested to the advantages of particular brands (testimonial ads were then becoming the rage in advertising strategies, used with all products and targeting men and women). Cigarette ads promoted adventure and social success with advertisements depicting smoking in a wide array of social and public settings.[65]

Cigarette manufacturer Lorillard introduced a new brand, Old Gold, around 1926 and, among other marketing efforts, hired artist John Held to draw his famous flapper girls for Old Gold ads. Around the same time a tiny company in the field of tobacco manufacturers, Philip Morris (it held just 0.5 percent of the cigarette market) positioned its Marlboro brand as a premium-priced smoke for women by putting it in a white pack with heavy foil, the royal crest in black and the slogan "The Mildness of America's best." Reinforcing the point were ads for the brand that prominently bore the phrase "Mild as May," the drawing of an obviously female hand holding a cigarette and a text that declared that no less outdated than the mustache cup, the overstuffed parlor, and the lapdog, was the

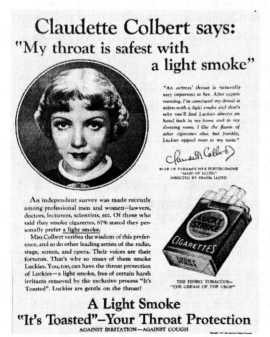

1937

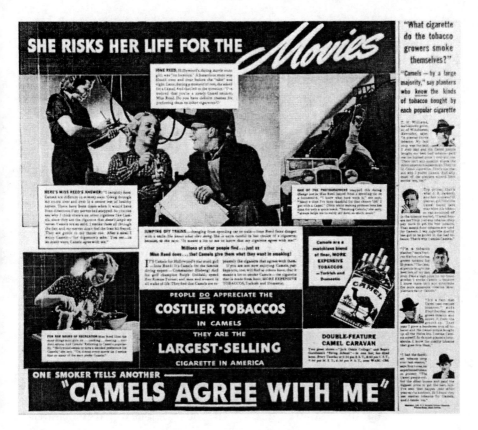

1938

notion that "decent, respectable women do not smoke.... Has smoking any
more to do with a woman's morals than has the color of her hair?" By 1927
Marlboro ads had become very direct in their pitches to women. They
read: "Women — when they smoke at all — quickly develop discerning
taste. That is why Marlboros ride in so many limousines, attend so many
bridge parties, repose in so many hand bags." To further pitch its smokes
to women Marlboro added an "ivory tip," a little laminated wrap around
the unlit end, to keep the cigarette paper from "clinging to lipsticked
mouths."[66]

Lucky Strike (American Tobacco) cigarettes entered the fray and
began targeting women, also in 1927. It solicited and printed testimonials
from European artists who informed the reader that they had discovered
their favorite cigarette in Lucky. A cigarette that was described as mild
and mellow because of a special process that treated the tobacco — "It's
Toasted." Luckies protected the user's throat, went the copy. American

Tobacco followed that up with more hard-hitting messages in their ads in 1928 and 1929 in which women were urged to smoke with the caption "Reach for a Lucky Instead of a Sweet." Backing up that campaign were testimonials from celebrities on the desirable effects on body weight and figure that could be achieved by substituting cigarettes for candy. Lucky ads hammered away at the importance of this image with ad headlines such as "Pretty Curves Win." In an ad headlined "The Grim Specter," a woman haunted by a double chin (seen in the shadow her face cast but not in her face itself—the shape of things to come) was urged, again, to reach for a Lucky instead. R. J. Reynolds (maker of Camel cigarettes) played it more cautiously. Its ads that year showed scenes of women alone, as well as in couples with a male, with the women getting closer and closer to actually smoking the cigarette. In the following year Reynolds ran an ad in which a woman offered a Camel to a man, who responded with a phrase that became legend, "I'd Walk a Mile for a Camel."[67]

Capturing the change that had taken place in some 18 months or less with respect to advertising cigarettes to women was Los Angeles reporter and columnist Alma Whitaker. In a column of April 14, 1929, she began by observing that "Slightly over a year ago we effulged in this column anent the fact that no cigarette advertiser had dared to depict a woman in any form of publicity." She also noted that the English advertisers had accepted the female cigarette smoker as a matter of course, that even advertisements for hats, clothing, sporting goods, and so on, showed females casually smoking cigarettes "and we virtuously rejoiced that the United States showed better taste in these matters." Whitaker reminded her readers that she went so far "as to deplore that American advertisers were edging closer to the idea ... showing us bill posters [billboards] with lovely, classy-looking maidens, enjoying, seemingly, a vicarious whiff from the smoke of the handsome male; or having some famous damsel remark that she preferred certain brands, although not

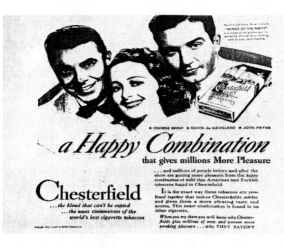

A trio of stars in 1939.

exactly admitting that she smoked 'em herself." In that earlier piece Whitaker also observed that an increasing number of women were smoking, but she approved of the fact they were not quite then "brazen" about it "and that even cigarette manufacturers were careful to respect the public attitude on the subject." But that was a year ago and those ads had changed drastically and dramatically. Females in the ads had moved from smiling benignly while a man held the pack, to her holding the pack, until "she was smoking 'em right out in public from billboards, in magazine and newspaper advertisements, in theater programs." She also mentioned the large number

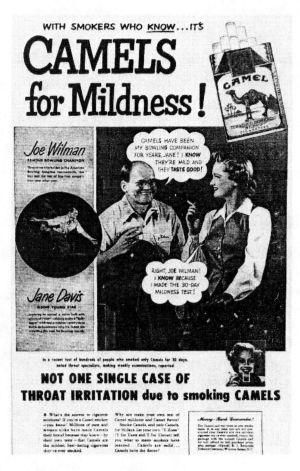

1949

of endorsement ads that suddenly appeared, from famous women endorsing various brands and "Once the spell against open confession was broken, it seemed that half the celebrated charmers were anxious to proclaim themselves addicts ... and probably found it very profitable to confess through those particular channels. According to Whitaker, the use of endorsement ads (using male and female celebrities) had increased the sales of cigarettes by some 33 percent in about one year.[68]

Endorsement ads, as mentioned, were very popular with many products in the late 1920s, and beyond, but especially so with cigarettes, with testimonial ads from male and female celebrities touting a particular smoke being especially prominent in the period starting around 1927 and continuing through the early 1950s. Many of them were phony. Early in 1927

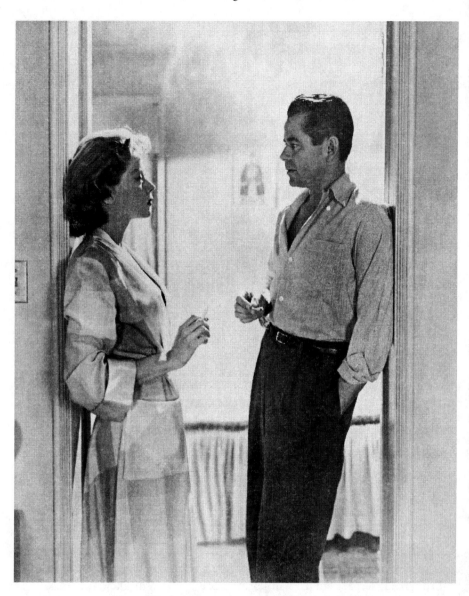

Gloria Grahame and Glenn Ford in *Human Desire*, 1954.

newspaper ads for Lucky Strike depicted opera star Ernestine Schumann-Heinke as using them regularly and as enjoying them during her leisure moments in her recently begun retirement. So distressed by this was the singer that she had placed the matter in the hands of an attorney. People she knew and did not know had mailed her copies of the ad and com-

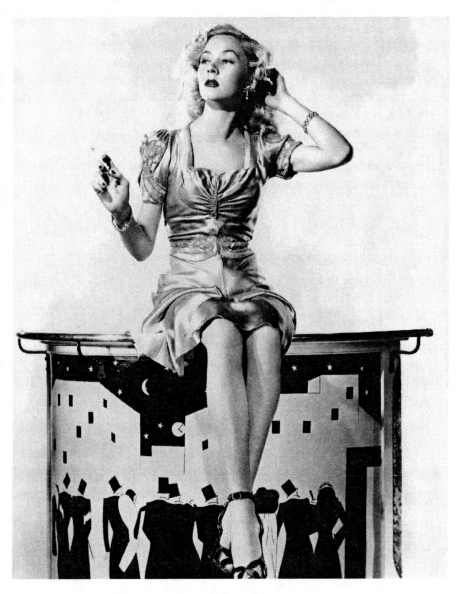

Gloria Grahame in a publicity shot ca. 1948.

mented negatively on her supposed use of the weed. "I have never smoked a cigarette in my life and, although I don't condemn women who do, neither do I approve of it in them," she exclaimed. Schumann-Heinke declared she had been made the victim of a hoax when her signature, reproduced at the bottom of the advertisement (which also contained her picture),

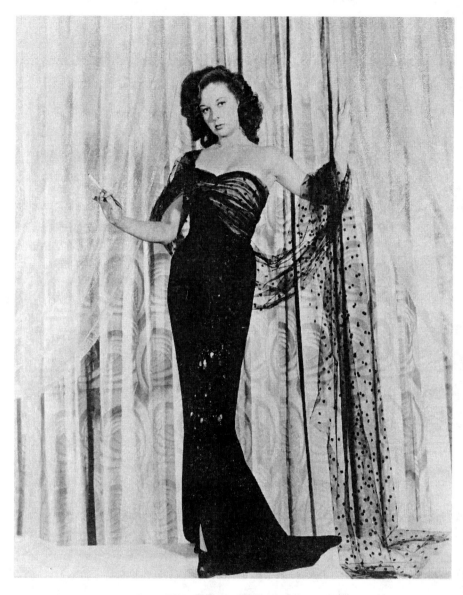

Susan Hayward in a publicity shot, 1940s.

was obtained. According to her, the son of a lifelong friend came to her several months earlier and told her she could help him make some money. With that story the young man readily obtained her signature to a note saying that she knew many American soldiers smoked that particular brand of cigarette in France. Instead of that indirect endorsement, however, the advertisement with her photo and signature told the world how the diva enjoyed smoking the cigarettes. Schumann-Heinke added, "My sons smoke and I worked four months during the war to raise money to buy cigarettes for the boys in France. But I never tasted one. Smoke would irritate my throat." (It was common for manufacturers of any product who wished to use an endorsement ad to use a middleman to approach the target celebrity. For example, an impoverished society women might have been approached by a cigarette marketer and asked to approach the target celebrity woman — to whom she was a friend or relative — to obtain the endorsement. In return the impoverished one would receive some sort of a fee if she were successful.) Her lawyer reportedly later obtained an injunction against the further appearance of that ad.[69]

Nor was that an isolated incident. During 1944 the Federal Trade Commission held hearings on a complaint charging the R.J. Reynolds Tobacco company with misleading advertising. Nothing came of the hearing, although information revealed that two women who signed testimonial ads in 1938 for Camel cigarettes were not regular smokers of that brand. Helen Stansbury, publicity director for Yardley of London, testified she had never smoked in her life (on three or four separate occasions she had experimented with one cigarette each time while a youth, but nothing beyond that), but admitted she received $100 for a Camel testimonial, which made it appear she smoked them. Noted photographer Margaret Bourke-White testified she received $250 for her endorsement and a weekly carton of Camels for a year. She declared she was "not an exclusive Camel smoker, although, frankly, I like Camels." Although complaints against several tobacco makers, all for alleged false advertising, were heard by the FTC in hearings that started in 1943 and traveled to several cities, and although apparently actionable facts turned up — such as the Stansbury admission — nothing happened.[70]

In the late 1920s as advertising campaigns were launched to attract more women to smoking there was also occurring all over the country a manifestation of the women's rights movement. Having recently won the right to vote, they were struggling for more, and perhaps starting to realize that the vote would not automatically solve all other problems for them. World War I was not long over, and when the men went to war the women were left at home to do both their jobs in the homes and those of the missing men in the factories. With the men back at home the women were expected to go quietly back to housework as if they had never been exposed to the financial and psychological independence which they had so recently enjoyed. For some women smoking had always been bound up with emancipation, freedom, and independence, the idea that men must never again be allowed to make general decisions that affected and controlled the lives of all women. Thus, by continuing to smoke, or by taking up the habit some women considered that action to be a statement, harking back to an independence one experienced in World War I, or harking forward as a result of suffrage — no more male control.

Another major figure in American advertising was Albert Lasker. He joined Chicago's Lord & Thomas ad agency in 1898. Later, Lasker and the American Tobacco Company's president, George Washington Hill, began working together to promote Lucky Strike cigarettes, in 1923; Lasker would promote Luckies until 1942. Reportedly Lasker's indignation over his wife being ordered not to smoke in a restaurant (apparently around 1923) led in a few years to that series of classic Lucky Strike magazine ads that directly targeted women. The notorious "Reach for a Lucky instead of a Sweet" campaign in 1928 had the confectionary industry up in arms. Lucky Strike remained Lasker's biggest account for about 15 years. His first ads, prior

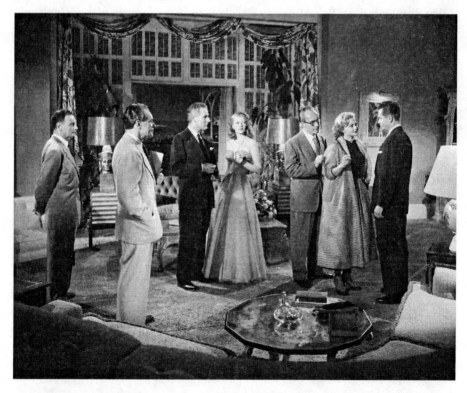

Rita Hayworth (with cigarette) and Glenn Ford (right) in *Affair in Trinidad*, 1952. Other cast members included Valerie Bettis, Walter Kohler (left), Karel Stepanek, Alexander Scourby (left center) and George Voscovek (wearing glasses).

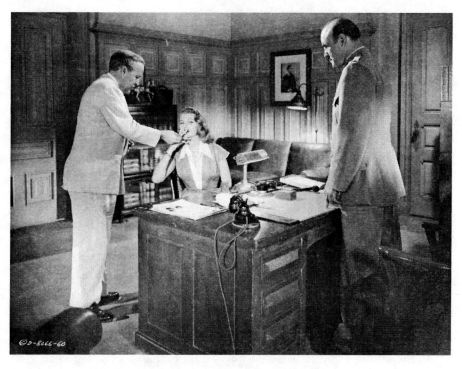

Rita Hayworth in *Affair in Trinidad*, 1952.

to 1927, directed toward women were also somewhat hesitant. One of his first featured a man smoking with a woman declaring, "I love the smell of a good cigarette." Later Lasker brought celebrities in to endorse the brand, depicting them as saying, "Lucky Strikes are soothing for the throat" and "I protect my precious voice thanks to Lucky Strike." Lasker was credited in this account for developing the campaign of using the new screen stars as Lucky endorsers, from the very late 1920s onward (the demand for movie stars as endorsers for any and all products went up sharply as the sophistication of the industry grew and especially upon the advent of sound films in 1927).[71]

A different account about some of the same ground eased Lasker out of the picture and eased Edward Bernays in. According to Allan Brandt's piece, in 1928 George Washington Hill turned his full attention to the problem of attracting women to the cigarette market. Soliciting the aid of public relations expert Bernays to help plan his strategy, Hill recognized the need to break the traditional social and cultural prohibitions against women smoking. In Bernays's words, "Hill became obsessed by the prospect of winning over the large potential female market for Luckies."

Hill enthused, "It will be like opening a new gold mine right in our own front yard." Advertising was to be just one crucial factor in what Bernays came to call "the engineering of consent." That effective manipulation of public opinion, interests, values and beliefs would in the 1920s become a dominant characteristic in the emergence of the consumer culture. After Hill and Bernays decided on the slogan, "Reach for a Lucky instead of a Sweet," they reportedly then set out to give meaning to that slogan. Recognizing that women's fashions were moving in the 1920s to a new emphasis on slimness, Lucky ads proclaimed the smoke to be a tool for achieving physical attractiveness and beauty. Said Brandt, "Bernays worked to influence the fashion industry, sending out hundreds of Parisian haute couture photos of slender models to fashion reporters and industry leaders."[72]

Brandt continued by saying that to strengthen his case Bernays cited medical writings on the negative impact of sugar on the human body. By 1929 Hill was said to have sought more aggressive intervention to change the meaning of women's smoking and to publicly attract that vast new market. Then Brandt outlined Bernays's version of the 1929 Easter Parade incident, including all the hype Bernays gave himself by describing it as of historic significance, setting off a national debate and, getting vast media coverage in all parts of America. The problem was, as noted earlier, none of those things seemed to have happened. Brandt added that cigarette ads targeted to women made explicit appeals to both beauty and style. In that period smoking for women became a part of the good life as defined in America's consumer culture. Through the images in the advertisements the symbolic meanings of glamour, beauty, autonomy, equality, and so on, were ascribed to the cigarette. Edward Bernays died in 1995, at the great age of 103. By the end of his life he had become active in the antismoking movement.[73]

Lucky Strike's campaign to smoke instead of eating candy to stay slim or become slim actually ran afoul of federal regulators and was brought to a halt. Early in 1930 the maker, American Tobacco, signed a consent order with the FTC in which it promised to stop using such phrases as "women retain slender figures" and "overweight is banished" in periodical, radio or other interstate advertising of its products. The regulator was upset because Lucky ads had featured "what purports to be the testimonials of famous people who smoked respondent's products and found they protect from irritation." Another complaint was that a Lucky ad had featured certain actresses in a musical show who were credited with the statement that because of Luckies "that's how we stay slender" when "in truth and in fact the said actresses were not cigarette smokers and did not stay slender through the smoking of respondent's cigarettes." Lucky Strike, concluded the FTC, used such advertising matter "when in truth and fact health and vigor to men, slender figures to women and reduction of flesh in all cases will not necessarily result from the smoking of respondent's brand of cigarettes." One of the reasons the FTC came down on Lucky Strike (and never at any time against any other maker, even though others acted similarly to American Tobacco) was that it alone had angered other powerful parts of the capitalist ruling order — the sugar trust, the candy lobby, and so on. Complaints from those powerful sectors of the overclass compelled the FTC to act.[74]

Starting in the very late 1920s, cigarette ads began to appear in major middle-class women's magazines such as *McCall's, Ladies Home Journal* and *Better Homes & Gardens*, directly pitching the product to women with ads

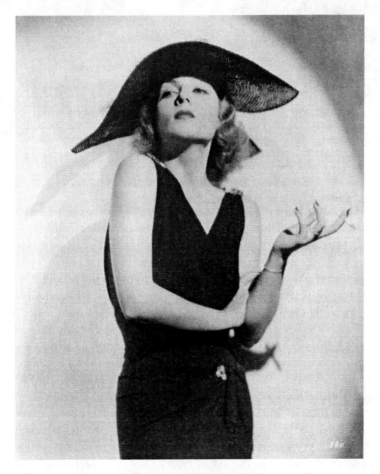

Carole Lombard in a publicity pose, ca. 1934.

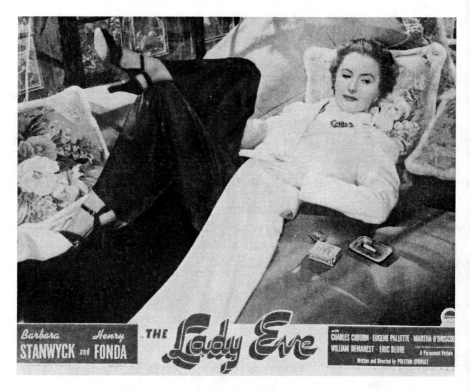

Barbara Stanwyck in *The Lady Eve*, 1941.

that featured testimonials from American female socialites (for Chesterfield cigarettes), and celebrities (Lucky Strike). Also, such ads featured elegant settings (during the Depression), athletic-appearing females, and women whose smoking made them sexually attractive. Cigarette brand preference of male and female smokers who responded to the 1938 *Fortune* magazine survey was "remarkably similar." An attempt by the Winston Cigarette Company at that time to market a cigarette called Fems, unique due to its red mouthpiece designed not to show lipstick marks, was not a success. Still, a 1937 survey of 500 people in four cities determined that 81 percent of the women interviewed did not approve of women smoking in public. By the time of World War II about one-third of U.S. women smoked cigarettes. During the war years, the ad campaigns of cigarette companies managed to link smoking with patriotism. Once again free packs of smokes were delivered to the armed forces, and in magazines women who smoked were depicted as role models who were hard at work in the national effort. However, the female smoker as a responsible and independent person ended with the war. During the second half of the 1940s in cigarette ads women were portrayed as wives and girlfriends, expecting or enjoying reunions with husbands and boyfriends returned from the war. One ad from the period featured a well-dressed couple looking out the window. The text read, "It's spring again. It's two again. Just the way it used to be. Two to grab for the morning paper. Two places to set at the table. And two Chesterfields over two cups of coffee."[75]

As might have been expected the sudden upsurge in tobacco ads aimed at women that began around 1927 and continued thereafter generated some angry opposition aimed at that particular aspect of the smoking women subject. National radio advertising by American Tobacco for its Lucky Strike brand that subtly advised women and other listeners that the way to retain health and shapely figures was to smoke plenty of cigarettes and go easy on food caused a vehement 1928 protest from the United Restaurant Owners' Association to be lodged with the Federal Radio Commission. Joseph Burger, president of the association, termed that cigarette advertising "insidious, unmoral and outrageous propaganda," and declared its purpose "apparently is to transform the school-girls and growing boys and youth of the country into confirmed cigarette addicts."[76]

F. M. Gregg, professor of education at Nebraska's Wesleyan University, said in 1929 that it was a recent boast of one of the tobacco trade journals that more women were then smoking than there were men smoking 20 years earlier. Persistent advertising and other forms of "propaganda" had brought the proportion of male smokers up to approximately seven or eight out of ten, so why not women in the same proportion? With that objective in mind, related Gregg, certain cigarette companies in the autumn of 1925 first introduced into their billboard advertisements the figure of an attractive woman, at first in company with a man, and later only the woman, and the inevitable pack of cigarettes. The face of the woman in those ads, thought Gregg, "is always marked by apparent purity and refinement" and "Still more recently the public has been compelled to see the embellished faces of famous artists of one kind or another, both male and female, along with a quoted indorsement of the particular brand of cigarettes advertised." When, wondered Gregg, would the cigarette be put into the woman's mouth in all the billboard advertisements? "It is already there on some billboards, on the stage, in the movie films, and all the magazines that are read by the feminine devotees of the cigarette," he reported. Worried such ads would soon be everywhere, Gregg explained,

> Now that enough women have already adopted the cigarette habit to make the practice rather common in certain public places, the attractive woman of the advertisements is beginning to carry a cigarette

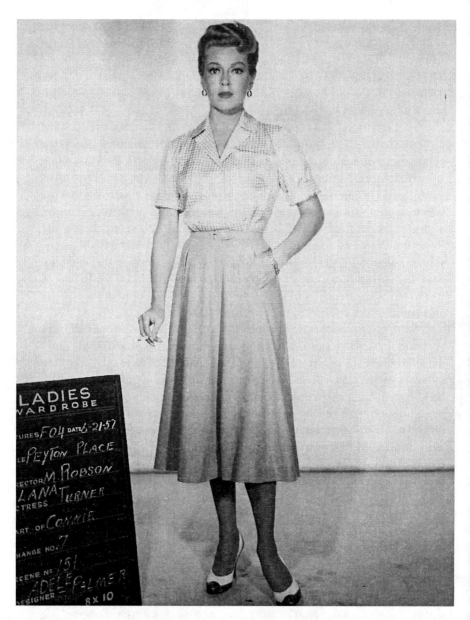

Lana Turner in a 1957 wardrobe shot.

between her own lips. The advertising policy of the cigarette companies has thus definitely hastened the day when this could happen without public protest. The ultimate objective has been achieved with amazing rapidity.[77]

Gregg said that at the time he was writing there were 35 million males who smoked, along with from 5 to 10 million females. That left some 25 million women yet to be drawn into the smoking habit, assuming equality was the goal of cigarette makers. With Americans then spending $3.6 billion per year on tobacco, if 25 million were added that would move total tobacco expenditure to $6 billion yearly, more than an adequate reason for marketers to practice "persistence in advertising." Gregg argued that an important contribution could be made by the women of America if by a widespread movement they should try to banish billboards from the landscape altogether. And, he suggested "through personal letters and by public protest the peculiarly insidious and vicious cigarette advertising carried on through the radio can be largely eliminated if all the people who are deeply disgusted and offended by it will only make themselves heard and felt through proper channels." As an example of a united effort to discourage or suppress all tobacco advertising that targeted women, Gregg cited 15 young people's societies in Ashland, Oregon, who were circulating an appeal to the local newspapers, the mayor, city council, and all advertising firms, asking them to oppose such advertising in all forms within the city limits. Their petition stated that such advertising "is contrary to the methods of thinking and living of Ashland youth, that the habit of using tobacco is unbecoming and degrading to any woman, and that they firmly believe American womanhood will stand for their convictions and ideals." A persistent campaign of such ads on billboards and radio in southern California aroused the opposition of the Glendale branch of the United Church Brotherhood of Los Angeles County. Deemed especially objectionable were the billboard advertisements. The Brotherhood, which had nearly 400 members, was appealing to county and city officials through its civics committee to suppress advertising of this nature. Gregg ended his piece with a dire warning: "It yet remains to be seen what a semiparalyzed public will actually do in the face of a menace that threatens to destroy the finer womanhood of America and permit the realization of that greatest menace to modern civilization, the complete masculinization of womankind."[78]

In May 1929, the Lodi (California) City Trustees ordered City Clerk Blakely to request a San Francisco billboard company to remove all its ads that featured cigarette-smoking females in a certain area of Lodi. Women's organizations in the community of Lodi had recently begun a movement against that type of advertising.[79]

Angered over the increasing numbers of advertisements designed to encourage cigarette smoking by women, delegates to the 33rd annual convention of the Western New York Federation of Women's Clubs meeting in Rochester, unanimously adopted a resolution protesting against ads "depicting women smoking or proffering lights." The measure, offered by federation executive Mrs. F. D. Turrentine, was directed to the attention of outdoor advertising firms that permitted such ads and to the leading officers of town and state. Meanwhile, in Sioux Falls, South Dakota, billboard ads that featured women smoking cigarettes so irked the city commission there that it voted, two to one, to forbid such things in Sioux Falls.[80]

Even as late as 1929, traditional views linking smoking with immorality lingered on. U.S. Senator Reed Smoot, in June of that year, introduced an unsuccessful bill in Congress to extend to tobacco the provisions of the Pure Food and Drugs Act of 1906. His remarks on the Senate floor revealed that the initial reluctance of the tobacco manufacturers to promote their product to women showed an awareness of the still prevalent sentiment,

> Not since the days when public opinion rose up in its might and smote the dangerous drug traffic, not since the days when the vendor of harmful nostrums was swept from our streets, has the country witnessed such an orgy of buncombe, quackery, and downright falsehood and fraud as now marks the current campaign promoted by certain cigaret manufacturers to create a vast woman and child market for the use of their product.[81]

Later in 1929, the *Christian Science Monitor* reprinted an editorial from a Plymouth, Massachusetts, publication, *Old Colony Memorial*. That latter publication condemned cigarette advertising directed at women and children using the same words uttered by Senator Smoot, without giving him credit. The editor added that in many women's colleges cigarettes had been distributed free by the manufacturers with the intention to start female undergraduates on the road to addiction. However, that was an allegation no one else had ever raised, and there was no other support for the claim. Urging both state and national legislative bodies to take action against such advertising, the editor demanded "the great untruths being spread by the printed word should be banned from distribution."[82]

Vigorous denunciations of the methods used by tobacco companies to increase cigarette smoking were made in December 1929 at the annual meeting of the Methodist Episcopal Church's Board of Temperance, Prohibition and Public Morals. Declaring the prohibition of tobacco was not intended, the board adopted a resolution protesting against the "exploitation of billboards of women smoking or in display advertising in magazines and newspapers" and on the radio. According to the resolution the practice was "subversive of essential racial interest and should be indignantly rebuked by American public sentiment."[83]

Renewing its attack against alleged false advertising of cigarettes early in 1930, the Board of Temperance, Prohibition and Public Morals, through its secretary, Dr. Clarence True Wilson, proposed that cigarette manufacturers be brought under the provisions of the federal Pure Food and Drugs Act. He believed that if the advertising of tobacco were to cease the number of tobacco users would likely drop by half in five years. "If the advertising directed to women ceased," added Wilson, "it is probable that within five years the smoking woman would be the rare exception." The policy of the American tobacco trust, he argued, seemed to be "to make such large advertising appropriations that they are able to purchase the support of athletes, popular heroes, society leaders, motion picture stars, and even medical men" and "to extend the use of tobacco to all women contrary to the fixed convictions and prejudices of the majority of American men." To control the industry, Wilson insisted it was necessary that the fraud be eliminated from cigarette advertising by subjecting the cigarette makers to he provisions of the Pure Food and Drugs Act. According to Wilson those tobacco manufacturers had once had to comply with that act, but "before the present offensive advertising policy of the tobacco manufacturers was adopted they sneaked out from under those provisions."[84]

14

The Opposition, 1927–1950

"Religious leaders among our women not only do not smoke but abhor the cigarette habit."
— *The Watchman-Examiner*, 1928

"So why not reach for a Bible instead of a smoke?"
— The Reverend Russell M. Brougher, 1929

General opposition to women smoking in this period disproportionately came from religious organizations and isolated individuals. It was weak, not well organized, and wholly unsuccessful. No laws remained on the books that were anticigarette statutes (excluding the ones prohibiting the sale of cigarettes to minors), and none were added. At an annual conference of the New Jersey Seventh Day Adventists in 1927 delegates were addressed by Dr. D. H. Kress, once the vice president of the Anti-Cigarette League and then acting medical secretary of the national organization of Adventists. Calling the cigarette habit one of the great dangers faced by the nation he said, "When smoking becomes as common among women as it now is among men there will be a landslide not only in physical and mental but also in moral degeneracy among their offspring." The habit also was at least a partial explanation of the rapidly decreasing birth rate in all civilized countries, he argued. Because of their more sensitive nervous system, Kress declared, "women take more readily than men to the soothing influence of the cigarette and it makes wrecks of them in time. Then, too, the cigarette smoker is not a home maker; she does not take kindly to domestic duties." Continuing on with his description of the smoking female Kress said, "she is nervous and restless, craving excitement. If children are born to her she will, in all probability, turn them over to others to be cared for. A child born to a cigarette smoker will, in time, become a nervous and mental wreck." As evidence, Kress cited conditions in Vienna

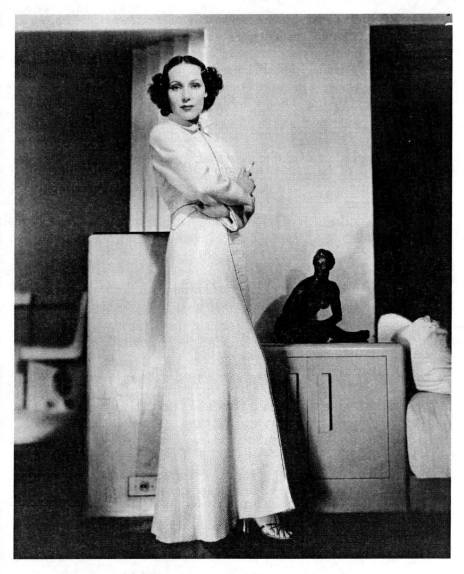

Dolores Del Rio in a publicity pose, ca. 1937.

"where smoking is prevalent among women," he said, as an example of the effects of the habit. Bizarrely, he then said that in 1926 there were 23,000 births and 26,000 deaths in that city while in Berlin deaths exceeded births by 289, with no further explanation.[1]

   One of the religious institutions heavily involved in the antismoking fight was the Methodist Episcopal Church. Maude Royden, famous English woman preacher, had a date to speak in Chicago in February 1928 under the auspices of the Woman's Home Missionary Society of the Methodist Episcopal Church, but her lecture was axed at the last minute. A rumor that Royden's fondness for smoking was responsible for the cancellation of the engagement by the Methodist women was denied by Mrs. Daniel Brummitt of Evanston, Illinois, in charge of the arrangements. Brummitt said it was simply a date conflict, that it could not use Royden on the date she had available. However, Brummitt insisted the visitor would speak in Chicago on the date arranged, just under the sponsorship of some other group, although she admitted she did not know what group that might be. When asked if there was any discussion in the organization concerning the fact Royden smoked, Brummitt evaded the point: "I think there is always more or less discussion wherever Miss Royden goes, about her smoking. It has been known, of course, for a long time, and it isn't as if it were a recent thing at all."[2]

A few days later when she was lecturing in Rochester, New York (on the same tour that was to have included Chicago), Royden answered a question in regard to cigarette smoking posed by Rochester women's groups. "Until the church bans smoking entirely among its male members, it is not in a very strong position to dictate what its women members should do about it," she said.[3]

The Royden affair quickly became well publicized, even covered in national media. Soon it became apparent that smoking did play a role in the affair. According to the New York *World*, the Chicago cancellation of the lecture was conveyed to Royden through a letter to William B. Feakins, manager of Royden's tour. Brummitt's letter stressed the alleged difference between the attitude toward smoking by women in the United States and in England by stating, "smoking is not a general practice in this country and is done not at all by the women of our churches." A subsequent statement was issued by Brummitt and sent out by the World Service Commission of the Methodist Episcopal Church. It said there was no knowledge on the part of the officers of the church at the time the lecture tour was arranged

> that Miss Royden had accepted the English custom of smoking. When the knowledge came, a conference was called of all general officers and chairmen of local committees, and it was decided that while, as American Christian women, they deprecated the practice, they could not presume to judge the integrity and the religious life of such a woman as Miss Royden, so it was decided to go ahead with arrangements.

But then, she added, local committees at Chicago and later Boston canceled their individual contracts, not the national body.[4]

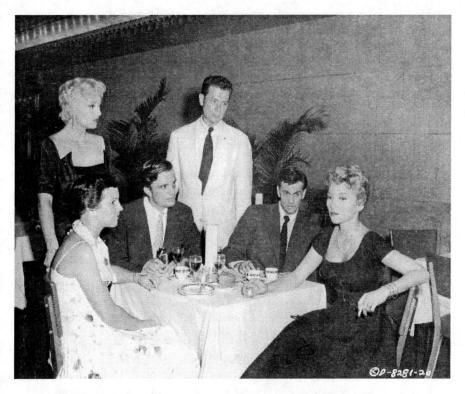

Beverly Garland (right) in *Riot on Pier Six*, 1955.

The furor generated much editorial comment, almost all of it in Royden's favor. Typical was the sentiment expressed by the Birmingham,
Alabama, *Age-Herald* that "if a lofty soul's right to be heard is to be judged
by whether a woman of flawless quality smokes, God help Chicago!" Said
the Washington, D.C., *Evening Star*, "To compare smoking with religion,
whether it is man or woman, is about as far-fetched as to say an automobile drive on Sunday afternoon is comparable to a safe-cracking job on
Sunday morning. Women, all classes and creeds, do smoke if they want
to, and it affects neither their morals nor their religion." In the words of
the New Haven *Register*,

> Assuredly no one in these days is going to stand forth and declare that
> because a woman indulges occasionally, or habitually, in cigaret smok-
> ing that she is any the less religious or that what she has to say on eth-
> ical matters of the hour is of any less importance. To attempt to link
> the smoking of cigarets with religion or ethics is so manifestly beneath
> the dignity of any organization of prominence or standing, that the effort
> merely reduces the argument to the level of child's play.[5]

One media outlet standing against Royden was *The Watchman-Examiner* (described as a leading Baptist journal), which declared it did not know the habits of England "but over here religious leaders among our women not only do not smoke but abhor the cigarette habit. By the example she is setting she is doing more harm than all the good she can do by address." In the opinion of this publication, when Royden learned the sentiment that existed in the United States, "she ought to have given up her cigarets instead of becoming an apologist for the cigaret habit among women."[6]

Controversy continued to dog Royden on her American tour, and in late February 1928, her scheduled visit to Santa Barbara, California, caused a rift in the Ministerial Union there. Royden was invited to speak there by the Reverend Oliver Hart Bronson, president of the Ministerial Union, but the Reverend Benjamin Goodfield of the First Baptist Church asserted the union had no part in bringing the cigarette-puffing evangelist to that city.

> I must clearly disassociate myself and my congregation in every way from any connection with the invitation recently extended to a Miss Maude Royden, a woman preacher of England, he stated. He said the notices in the area papers of her lecture gave the impression she was coming to Santa Barbara under the auspices of the Ministerial Union and that she is consequently endorsed by them. This is entirely wrong.

However, she was defended by the Reverend Paul A. Davies of the First Congregational Church: "No minister in Santa Barbara especially commends her for indulgence in tobacco, but some of us cannot let an occasional cigarette hide her sterling qualities of Christian character, her able preaching of vital Christianity, nor the tremendous results of her work."[7]

One year later Dr. Clarence True Wilson, secretary of the Methodist Episcopal Board of Temperance and Morals, gave a lecture in the Arcadia Auditorium in Washington, D.C., on the topic of "The Deadly Cigarette." Declared Wilson, "We are not fanatical on the subject, but the time has come for Congress to wipe out the lying, murderous campaign of the American Tobacco Trust and for us to teach these conscienceless baby-killers a lesson that will live for a generation." Grumbling about the pervasiveness of cigarette advertising, Wilson decried in particular that which was directed at women and children. About a year earlier, he said, the tobacco "trust began to enter the field of American women and children with advertising. First women were shown in groups where there was smoking. Then cigarettes were shown in feminine hands, and finally women were urged by advertising and radio to substitute the cigarette for sweets." A reporter observed that the entry of the Methodist organization into the anticigarette arena followed the lead of similar campaigns of food and candy organizations making a drive to keep programs sponsored by cigarette makers off the air, which, however, had made no headway with the Federal Radio Commission.[8]

Still not finished, the Methodist Episcopal Board of Temperance announced in 1931 that it was launching a joint attack on the tobacco companies and on manufacturers of grape concentrates fermentable into wine. Condemned by the board was the creation of an "impression that the use of cigarettes by young women is socially necessary" and the testimony "bought" from physicians and others concerning the effects of tobacco (referring to paid endorsement ads). Added the board, "The tobacco companies stand convicted of profiteering in the flesh and blood of unborn children."[9]

Religious attacks on smoking women were not limited to the Methodist organization. The Reverend Russell M. Brougher delivered an address in 1929 in the Baptist Temple, Brooklyn. It was in response to a request for sermons on dry law enforcement by the Brooklyn WCTU, but he also attacked cigarette smoking. With respect to the rapid spread of the habit among American women, he fumed that it was "not only the greatest single degenerative influence among our people, but is also an influence which more than any other threatens the integrity of our civilization.... So why not reach for a Bible instead of a smoke?"[10]

Representative delegates attending the National Students Leadership convention in Chicago in 1929 (all the delegates were men from Catholic colleges) were of the opinion that the females of America in 1929 did not get the respect that gentlemen paid their gender a few years earlier. And that was because "they offend the conventions so much." With respect to the woman who smoked cigarettes, Joseph Doran (Fordham University, New York) said, "It gets her fingers all stained up." Donald J. Ranney (John Carroll University, Cleveland) declared, "The trouble is she's likely to offend some one." J. Francis Walsh (Loyola University, Chicago) commented, "So many of them start smoking because they want to be 'good fellows.' Anyway, that's what they say. But why should they want to be good fellows, or any other kind of fellows? They never were and never will be. They ought to be themselves." Ranney added that if the women wanted more respect, "they should drop some of their free and easy ways." Doran also said, "Now, it may be that a girl walking down the streets with a backless dress and no stockings—smoking a cigarette in the bargain—is an extremely moral young woman. But when folks look at her they don't think so. They think otherwise. The average man figures she isn't respectable and consequently he doesn't treat her with respect." All those men started off by telling the reporter that they did not see anything wrong in a female smoking and then added the caveats.[11]

A resolution condemning smoking among women, especially Catholic college women, was adopted in 1931 by the college section of the National Catholic Educational Association at its annual meeting. Sister Mary Aloysius, head of the College of St. Teresa (Verona, Minnesota), deplored the prevalence of smoking among college women and asserted that, while the church recognized that smoking was not a sin, the Catholic college girl who smoked, especially while attending a school conducted by nuns, provided a bad influence for others.[12]

Nonreligious individuals and groups were not absent from the assault. Even the Boy Scouts became involved briefly. As of July 1928, the 6,000 Boy Scouts of Cleveland had a new "daily good turn" to add to their opportunities. A resolution passed by the executive committee of the Boy Scout Council, and said to be for "psychological reasons," admonished each scout to use his influence to stop cigarette smoking by women. Scout executives explained the boys would approach women they came across smoking in public, asking them to give up the weed. A spokesperson for the national headquarters of the Boy Scouts (based in New York) said that if the Cleveland scouts were conducting a campaign there to curb smoking by women, it was without the knowledge of the national headquarters. All such projects, observed the spokesperson, had to receive the sanction of the central body before they were put into effect. Cleveland Boy Scout executives explained they felt "smoking coarsens them and detracts from the ideal of fine motherhood."[13]

An editor for the *New York Times* brought up an obvious problem for the Cleveland scouts' plan — regarding the final taboo, which had not then fallen completely — when he wondered, "But how will they know, by passing women in the streets, whether they smoke? It is not customary to see women smoking in the streets."[14]

Within a week the action of the Executive Committee of the Cleveland Boy Scout Council in their plan to create a sentiment against smoking by women by "the million Boy Scouts of our country," had been formally repudiated by the Executive Board of the Boy Scouts of America. In a letter to Floyd A. Rowe, president of the Cleveland Boy Scout Council, James E. West, chief scout executive, took the Cleveland body to task for acting in a manner that was not in the province of a local council and that involved "misunderstanding as to the real aims and purposes of the Boy Scout movement." West stated the movement sought to instill habits of good character in boys, but it did not intend to lead Boy Scouts to interfere in the private concerns of individuals. That repudiated resolution adopted by the Executive Committee declared,

Be it resolved that whereas recent advertisements have been creeping closer and closer toward the inducement of girls to adopt the smoking of cigarettes, and whereas this purpose is being more and more plainly announced, it is felt to be the duty of this council to declare that the now-appearing billboard advertisement which portrays a young lady reading a letter to the effect that girls who seek pleasure in smoking are flocking to that given brand of cigarette, is an advertisement which merits strong disapproval and censure, because it is a flagrant luring and seductive effort to entice the girlhood of America to the habit of smoking. We commend to each of the million Boy Scouts of our country that he adopt as his "daily good turn" the creation of a sentiment disapproving of such unpatriotic efforts as the enticement of our girls and young men."[15]

An editorial insert into a 1929 article not favorable toward female cigarette smoking had the editor of this magazine declare, "*Good Housekeeping* is just old-fashioned enough to wish that women would not smoke.... And *Good Housekeeping* objects to the way in which cigarettes are being advertised"— that is, endorsement ads by celebrities.[16]

From Boston at the end of 1930 came an announcement that a newly organized antismoking league for women planned a nationwide drive against smoking, except by grown men. In other words it was only going to target women and children. Plans called for the aid of women's clubs and organizations, and schools to be enlisted as well as to flood the country with circulars, posters and stickers. Storekeepers were to be monitored, and any who sold cigarettes to minors were to be reported to the authorities. Additionally, the cooperation of officials of high schools and girls' colleges would be sought. Alexander Rice (of Dorchester, Massachusetts), financial backer of the new league and father-in-law of Eleanor Rice, its treasurer, said the group would conduct a campaign of education and would not seek any prohibitory legislation. Nothing more was heard from that proposed organization.[17]

Glassboro, New Jersey's Board of Education produced a code for

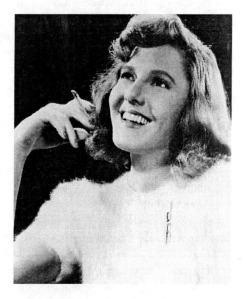

Jean Arthur in *The Devil and Miss Jones,* 1941.

the personal conduct of its schoolteachers at the start of the 1933-34 school year and sent that order to all of its teachers, "most of them young women." Among other items, the code advised teachers "to have regard for the preponderance of local public opinion against smoking by women." The board warned that although it "respected" the rights of individual freedom, dismissal awaited any teacher "whose reputation for personal conduct may to any degree be considered detrimental to the desired influence of the teacher in the school or community."[18]

When Anna Steese Richardson, editor and "leader" of women's activities, delivered an address to the Women's Advertising Club of Detroit in 1935, she exclaimed, "I'm fed up with this cigarette smoking. It isn't the smoking I object to, but women are so darned rude about it. I'd like to go into a washroom on a Pullman just once and not find ashes all over the washbowl." In a more wide-ranging diatribe she added, "Women are getting uglier every day. Women diet until they look haggard, and then they wear low-backed dresses which show the little chain of bones down their backs. I wonder how any of them ever got a man."[19]

Mrs. Lloyd W. Biddle, president of the Federation of Women's Clubs, in a 1937 address lashed out by saying, "Smoking in public is one of the most vicious habits women have today and makeup in public is awful, especially for the example of our daughters." She also denounced drinking by women before concluding, "women should hold the banner of womanhood so high that they would be put back on the pedestal they occupied before the war. The race rises no higher than its women."[20]

A 1938 piece in Reader's Digest attacked women smokers on the grounds of bad form, smoking and eating together, for example, and never having mastered the art of smoking "properly,"— that is, female puffers had too many "conspicuous affectations." Men had none of those problems, went the piece. Also women, unlike men, were discourteous smokers because they never asked permission before lighting up and scattered ashes everywhere. Concluded the piece, "Women don't and probably never will understand the philosophy and ideal of good form that men have developed as regards the use of tobacco. They're not even amateurs, bless them. They're comedians."[21]

One of the last of the old-time attacks on smoking women — and it was very late because such attacks pretty much disappeared around the mid–1930s— was delivered in 1950 by AFL Teamsters Union President Daniel J. Tobin (a former smoker) who declared that smoking was bad for everybody, especially women. Not only did it damage health, he also thought it was dangerous to a female's moral standing. Writing in his union's monthly magazine, the Teamster, Tobin said he knew that "mil-

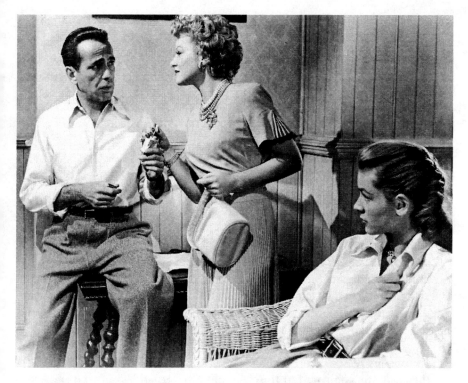

Humphrey Bogart, Claire Trevor, and Lauren Bacall (right) in *Key Largo*, 1948.

lions of wonderful young, noble women do smoke," but he did not believe "it adds to their moral standing or to the respect that men may hold for them." Most disgusting of all to Tobin was to see a 50-year-old woman walking down the street "with a cigarette hanging in her lips without even holding same in her hand and not endeavoring to hide it."[22]

15

Conclusion

Around the mid– to late–1800s, women began the long struggle to break the male domination of society and establish themselves as people with all the rights and responsibilities that were accorded to men — to be equal citizens. Women could not vote, or work in many of the professions, and so on. Males had decided for females just what places the latter would hold in society, and they were very limited. Among the many things women strived for was the right to smoke, outside the home, the way that men did. As the 1900s began, men could smoke just about anywhere outside the home, while women could smoke almost nowhere. Women had to overcome male and female opposition to their gender taking up the habit, for various reasons, and to overcome the opposition that existed against the cigarette, compared to the cigar and pipe, regardless of who smoked it. But the cigarette was destined to dominate as the favored form of tobacco consumption mainly because improved production methods had made it much more convenient and much less expensive than any of its rivals.

European women led the way in the period 1880–1908 when the issue of female smoking began to capture public and media attention. Prior to 1880 there was very little tobacco consumption by females. By 1908, the custom of women smoking had achieved very widespread acceptance abroad, especially in the United Kingdom; it was not uncommon for women to be seen smoking in restaurants, cafés, and women's clubs. In America, though, things were quite different. Through that period there was no smoking by women allowed in any public places such as restaurants, trains, hotel common areas, and so on. But it did take place, and more women turned to the habit. They smoked at home and at dinners, parties, and other gatherings of the upper classes. For in the United States and abroad it was the upper-class women who did most of the smoking, or so accounts claimed. Either the lower-class women hardly indulged or it drew no comment. From the fashionable set in America, the cigarette smoking habit spread downward to the other social classes.

All smoking in America was covert in this period. It was so hidden that reporters— seeking to quantify the situation — were unable to produce any numbers and had to rely on indirect and anecdotal evidence to support the idea that more women were smoking. Hairdressers, manicurists, dentists, doctors, and so on, were cited as relating that more of their female clients and patients had tobacco-stained fingers and cigarette breath. One of the strongest taboos involving women and smoking was the idea that a female did not smoke in the street. Such an act could cause a woman to run afoul of the police and even face the possibility of jail time.

A strong opposition movement against smoking was active in this period, led by women and women's groups. The idea of the time that women were far more moral, decent, clean-living, respectable, and so on, than were men, led to them being condemned all the more for the practice while also making them the logical choice to lead the opposition. Organized, vocal, persistent, and belligerent, that opposition was very successful in the sense that it caused a lot of laws to be placed on a lot of statute books; most of those laws banned the sale of smokes to minors, but some of them barred the sale of cigarettes to all, including adults. In another sense those laws were unsuccessful because they were rarely (if ever), enforced. Avoiding the antagonizing of males (most of them usually smoked cigars, and pipes to a lesser extent) most of those opposition campaigns targeted boy smokers and female puffers (almost all of them used cigarettes) with most of the enacted laws banning the sale of cigarettes but not other forms of tobacco, such as cigars, pipe tobacco, and so on.

During the period 1908–19 in America, a huge change took place. For one thing, the lowly cigarette had almost had its image completely rehabilitated and still more women were recruited to the habit. Women took the issue of smoking in public to restaurants and hotel common areas. Many confrontations and awkward moments took place in such establishments over this period. In 1908 virtually no restaurants in America officially allowed women to smoke in their general dining areas. By 1919 most of them allowed the practice, driven to change by pressure from their customers. The shift from a mostly no to a mostly yes environment began around 1912–13. Nor was such a change limited to New York City, which might have been expected to lead the way in such a matter. Women smoked in the restaurants and hotels of other cities such as San Francisco, Los Angeles, Washington, and Chicago. Some vaudeville theaters added smoking rooms for women to their venues. Still, many public places remained off limits to female puffers, such as trains, stores, and especially the open street. Jail time was still handed out to women audacious enough to puff openly. Also, the fact that a woman smoked could be (and was), used in court as a negative marker, a cause to reinforce a case that she was insane, that she was not fit to have custody of her children, and so forth. Opposition movements were weakened by the rehabilitation of the cigarette's image but strengthened by constitutional amendments that gave women the vote and banned alcohol nationwide. Hurling the epithet of "smoker" at a woman could still stigmatize her. Individuals were often singled out for attacks, ostensibly for the bad example they set, such as Alice Roosevelt Longworth. Ellen Wilson, wife of candidate Woodrow Wilson, felt compelled to publicly denounce a rumor she was a closet smoker as false during Woodrow's successful campaign for president.

With respect to women and smoking in America in the period 1919–27, the dominant focus was on the issue of whether women students in colleges and universities should smoke, and if so, where. Almost no such institution allowed its women students to indulge in 1920; by 1925 most permitted the practice, albeit often with restrictions. With cigarettes sweeping the campuses (Bryn Mawr reported 45 percent of its student body were smokers) another major step had been taken toward the acceptance of the custom in society. Young women, members of the intelligentsia and future leaders within female society, had won the right to smoke and enthusiastically took to the cigarette. More and more public places allowed the smoking woman — railroads, more theaters, street railway systems, and so on. The only taboo that more or less held fast was that women still did not smoke in the street. Negative consequences still resulted from such behavior. Opposition to smoking, in any organized fashion, had disappeared from America by 1927. The old-style attacks whereby women badgered and hectored young boys on the street and legislators in state capitols, had fallen out of fashion by this time. More and more the opposition was reduced to isolated individuals and weak groups. Increasingly the opposition was seen as eccentrics and cranks. Symbolically, the last law on the books that banned sales to adults was repealed in 1927 (it had never been enforced to any extent). A few cities thought about enacting bylaws to ban women from smoking in public places such as restaurants, but got nowhere in the wake of female suffrage and the blatant discrimination inherent in such proposals. The time for such laws was over.

During the final period, 1927–50, smoking by women spread everywhere — to hairdressers, to department stores, and even to the street, as that last taboo fell sometime in the 1930s. A major issue of this period was the use of advertising by cigarette makers that targeted women directly. Prior to 1927 there was next to no advertising of cigarettes aimed directly or indirectly at women. Statistics on the number of women who smoked in the time period covered by this book were not available. For the period prior to 1927 or so, there were not even educated estimates. For 1929–31 it was estimated that women consumed 12–14 percent of cigarettes sold; for 1935 another source put the female smoking rate at 18 percent; another said the figure was 33 percent in 1949. What opposition remained active in this period was even weaker and more marginalized than in the past.

As the innocent years drew to a close, around 1950, women were accepted as smokers to the same extent that men were and in the same places. Of course, the years 1880–1950 were not completely innocent. Many medical reports had come out within that period pointing out the health hazards of smoking. For whatever reason, though, they had been largely ignored. Very early in the 1950s an increased number of reports came out, reinforcing the link between the habit and lung cancer, heart disease, and other ills. Still later in the 1950s, some public places barred smoking. That was a significant reversal because from 1880 onward the history of smoking had been one of more and more public places allowing the practice, first to men and then to women. By the 1950s, then, the cigarette had begun its return journey, back to regaining the pariah status it had held less than 50 years earlier. As the 1950s began, although it was not then clear, the smoking party was definitely over for everybody.

Notes

Chapter 1

1. Alfred Dunhill. "The woman's pipe." *Times* (London), October 20, 1925, tobacco supp., p. 21.
2. G. L. Apperson. *The Social History of Smoking*. London: Martin Secker, 1914, pp. 208–10.
3. *Ibid.*, pp. 210–15.
4. *Ibid.*, pp. 215–20.
5. "The Victorian days." *Times* (London), December 30, 1926, p. 6.
6. "The Victorian days." *Times* (London), January 3, 1927, p. 8; "The Victorian days." *Times* (London), January 1, 1927, p. 6; "The Victorian days." *Times* (London), January 4, 1927, p. 6.
7. Cassandra Tate. *The Triumph of the Little White Slaver*. New York: Oxford University Press, 1999, pp. 22–23.
8. "Women who smoke rare." *New York Times*, December 9, 1894, p. 18.
9. Tate, op. cit., p. 24.
10. "From snuff to cigarettes." *Washington Post*, March 26, 1906, p. 6.
11. "The use of tobacco." *New York Times*, September 14, 1874, p. 3.
12. "Use of snuff increasing." *Los Angeles Times*, February 11, 1899, p. 7.

Chapter 2

1. Eunice Fuller Barnard. "The cigarette has made its way up in society." *New York Times*, June 9, 1929, pp. SM6, SM18.
2. "Smoking history and background." Online document, www.webspawner.com/users/smokingbackground, January 2004.
3. Ronald J. Troyer and Gerald E. Markle. *Cigarettes: The Battle Over Smoking*. New Brunswick, New Jersey: Rutgers University Press, 1983, pp. 34–35.
4. *Ibid.*, p. 40.
5. "Smoking history and background," op. cit.
6. Richard Kluger. *Ashes to Ashes*. New York: Alfred A. Knopf, 1996, p. 62.
7. Virginia L. Ernster. "Mixed messages for women." *New York State Journal of Medicine* 85 (July 1985): 335.
8. Jacob Sullum. *For Your Own Good: The Anti-Smoking Crusade and the Tyranny of Public Health*. New York: Free Press, 1998, p. 28.

Chapter 3

1. "The use of tobacco." *New York Times*, September 14, 1874, p. 3.
2. "Women and smoking." *New York Times*, September 1, 1879, p. 2.
3. "Women who smoke." *Washington Post*, November 4, 1888, p. 9.
4. "Women and home." *Los Angeles Times*, March 30, 1893, p. 10.
5. "Society women smoking." *Washington Post*, July 16, 1893, p. 12.
6. "Shall women smoke?" *Los Angeles Times*, November 13, 1893, p. 4.
7. "Women and tobacco." *New York Times*, February 28, 1897, p. SM5; "Use of cigarettes." *Los Angeles Times*, April 1, 1897, p. 8.
8. "Smoking women augment." *New York Times*, March 6, 1898, p. 7.

9. "London women smoke in public." *Los Angeles Times*, November 26, 1899, p. 30.

10. "Fashion's frivolities." *Weekly Dispatch* (UK), February 25, 1900, p. 15.

11. "Die then, and smoke, said his majesty." *Los Angeles Times*, June 28, 1901, p. 1.

12. "London's women smokers." *Washington Post*, February 23, 1902, p. 34.

13. Elizabeth L. Banks. "English women smoke cigarettes." *Washington Post*, October 26, 1902, p. 19.

14. "Where woman shares man's joy in pipe and cigar." *Washington Post*, July 30, 1905, p. B5.

15. "Smoking car for women." *New York Times*, March 22, 1906, p. 1.

16. Elizabeth Biddle. "Cigarette smoking among Englishwomen no uncommon practice." *New York Times*, March 25, 1906, p. SM7.

17. *Ibid.*

18. "Lady smokers of England." *Los Angeles Times*, July 8, 1906, sec. 1, p. 6.

19. *Ibid.*

20. "Bars bridge and smoking." *New York Times*, July 23, 1907, p. 4.

21. "Many women are smokers." *Los Angeles Times*, January 5, 1908, sec. 1, p. 4.

Chapter 4

1. "Tiny pipes for women." *Washington Post*, July 8, 1888, p. 12.

2. "Women who smoke." *Washington Post*, November 25, 1888, p. 12.

3. "Feminine smokers." *Washington Post*, March 2, 1890, p. 15.

4. "Cigarette-smoking women." *Washington Post*, February 1, 1891, p. 4.

5. Mrs. M'Guirk. "Lady cigarettes." *Los Angeles Times*, March 18, 1894, p. 15.

6. *Ibid.*

7. "Women who smoke rare." *New York Times*, December 9, 1894, p. 18.

8. "Society's new woman." *Washington Post*, June 2, 1895, p. 14.

9. "Dainty cigarettes for women." *Washington Post*, December 15, 1895, p. 20.

10. "Cigarettes and fair fingers." *Washington Post*, February 16, 1896, p. 22.

11. Helen Bullitt Lowry. "To smoke or not to smoke." *New York Times*, June 26, 1921, sec. 7, pp. 2, 9.

12. Jacob Sullum. *For Your Own Good: The Anti-Smoking Crusade and the Tyranny of Public Health.* New York: Free Press, 1998, p. 35.

13. "Women cigarette smokers." *New York Times*, June 24, 1901, p. 7.

14. "Smokers among the fair sex." *Washington Post*, February 28, 1904, p. A8.

15. Julian Hawthorne. "Can ladies smoke tobacco?" *Washington Post*, October 25, 1903, p. F3.

16. Marie Studholme. "Should women smoke?" *Washington Post*, October 2, 1904, p. B3.

17. Alexander Barton. "Should women smoke?" *Washington Post*, October 2, 1904, p. B3.

18. "Cigarette habit growing among Washington women?" *Washington Post*, April 1, 1906, p. E6.

19. "Cigarette habit grips women." *Los Angeles Times*, September 22, 1907, sec. 7, p. 6.

20. *Ibid.*

21. "Delmonico bars women smokers." *Los Angeles Times*, October 22, 1897, p. 14.

22. "Smokers among the fair sex." *Washington Post*, February 28, 1904, p. A8.

23. "The women who smoke." *New York Times*, December 3, 1897, p. 8.

24. "Smoked 1907 out." *Washington Post*, January 1, 1908, p. 1.

25. "Not all may smoke." *Washington Post*, January 5, 1908, p. 10.

26. *Ibid.*

27. *Ibid.*

28. "She smoked on the Avenue." *Washington Post*, December 29, 1895, p. 2.

29. "Women and cigarettes." *Washington Post*, December 30, 1895, p. 6.

30. "May women smoke in auto?" *New York Times*, September 26, 1904, p. 1.

31. "The use of tobacco." *New York Times*, September 14, 1874, p. 3.

32. "Women and smoking." *New York Times*, September 1, 1879, p. 2.

33. "Should women smoke?" *Washington Post*, March 6 1892, p. 12.

34. "Society women smoking." *Washington Post*, July 16, 1893, p. 12.

35. "Smokers among the fair sex." *Washington Post*, February 28, 1904, p. A8.

36. "Advises women to smoke." *New York Times*, August 27, 1906, p. 1.

37. "Woman with tobacco heart." *Los Angeles Times*, March 7, 1907, sec. 1, p. 14.

Chapter 5

1. "Varieties." *News of the World* (UK), June 20, 1886, p. 6.
2. "Will the coming woman smoke?" *Los Angeles Times*, August 20, 1893, p. 12.
3. "Smoking: online exhibits." Kansas State Historical Society, Online document, www.kshs.org, January 2004.
4. *Ibid.*
5. "Advanced woman upheld." *New York Times*, September 2, 1895, p. 5.
6. "Women using narcotics." *New York Times*, January 10, 1897, p. 13.
7. "Online exhibits: Carry A. Nation." Kansas State Historical Society, Online Document, www.kshs.org, January 2004.
8. *Ibid.*
9. "Smoking: online exhibits," op. cit.
10. "Cigarettes fashionable?" *Los Angeles Times*, April 19, 1906, sec. 2, p. 13.
11. *Ibid.*
12. Cassandra Tate. *The Triumph of the Little White Slaver.* New York: Oxford University Press, 1999, p. 24.
13. Allan M. Brandt. "Recruiting women smokers: the engineering of consent." *Journal of the American Medical Women's Association* (January–April 1996); p. 63.
14. Tate, op. cit., p. 23.
15. "Stop smoking them, boys." *Washington Post*, November 24, 1890, p. 8.
16. "The history of tobacco, part II (1700–1899)." History Net, Online Document, www.historian.org, January 2004.
17. "Under W.C.T.U. ban." *New York Times*, May 18, 1907, p. 6.
18. Jarrett Rudy. "Unmaking manly smokers: church, state, governance, and the first anti-smoking campaigns in Montreal, 1892–1914." *Journal of the Canadian Historical Association* 12 (2001): 95, 109–110.
19. *Ibid.*, p. 110.
20. *Ibid.*, pp. 111–114.
21. Frances Warfield. "Lost cause." *Outlook and Independent* 154 (February 12, 1930): 244.
22. Meta Lander. *The Tobacco Problem*, 6th ed. 1882; Boston: Lee and Shepard, 1899, p. 29.
23. Warfield, op. cit., pp. 244–45.
24. *Ibid.*, p. 245.
25. Gordon L. Dillow. "Thank you for not smoking." *American Heritage* 32 (February/March 1981): 102.
26. Warfield, op. cit., p. 245.
27. *Ibid.*, pp. 245–46.

28. "Women and cigarettes." *Washington Post*, March 29, 1906, p. A1.
29. Warfield, op. cit., p. 246; "Miss Gaston begins anti-cigarette war." *New York Times*, September 12, 1907, p. 2.
30. Jacob Sullum. *For Your Own Good: The Anti-Smoking Crusade and the Tyranny of Public Health.* New York: Free Press, 1998, pp. 30–31.
31. Dillow, op. cit., pp. 102–104.

Chapter 6

1. "Czarina forbids smoking." *Los Angeles Times*, February 18, 1908, sec. 2, p. 4.
2. "Women smoke less." *Washington Post*, November 29, 1908, p. 17.
3. "Women abuse the weed." *New York Times*, May 21, 1913, p. 3.
4. "To reform Paris also." *New York Times*, June 21, 1908, p. C2.
5. "Shall women smoke?" *Los Angeles Times*, October 31, 1908, sec. 2, p. 4.
6. "Scoff at W.C.T.U." *Washington Post*, August 21, 1910, p. 9.
7. "Disobeying Queen Mary." *Los Angeles Times*, May 14, 1911, pp. 1–2; "Duchess smokes cigars." *Washington Post*, December 21, 1913, p. 1.
8. Alma Whitaker. "My lady nicotine." *Los Angeles Times*, October 23, 1912, sec. 2, p. 6.
9. "Milady puffs cigars." *Washington Post*, March 22, 1914, p. 2.
10. "Fair smokers' mecca." *Washington Post*, April 5, 1914, p. 4.
11. "English women smoke too much." *Los Angeles Times*, May 9, 1917, sec. 2, p. 1.
12. "Girl's smoking record." *Washington Post*, September 19, 1917, p. 6.
13. Marion Ryan. "All the men and women merely wills's." *Weekly Dispatch* (UK), November 25, 1917, p. 4.
14. *Ibid.*
15. "The cigarette hoarders." *Weekly Dispatch* (UK), December 9, 1917, p. 3.
16. "The field is the world." *New York Times*, February 13, 1919, p. 14.

Chapter 7

1. "Newport to war on smoking by women." *New York Times*, May 3, 1908, p. 11.

2. "Smoking among women." *Washington Post*, July 30, 1911, p. E4.

3. "Assert women are smokers." *Los Angeles Times*, October 28, 1912, p. 3.

4. "Puffs rings of smoke while taking the air." *Los Angeles Times*, December 7, 1912, p. 1.

5. "Women's cigarette holders." *Los Angeles Times*, December 8, 1912, sec. 3, p. 25.

6. "Smoking on increase here." *Washington Post*, December 19, 1912, p. 4.

7. "Objects to women smoking." *New York Times*, January 11, 1913, p. 1.

8. "Would tar Stotesbury." *Washington Post*, January 13, 1913, p. 1.

9. "King's ransom goes in smoke." *Los Angeles Times*, December 19, 1914, sec. 2, pp. 1, 6.

10. "One woman in Chicago of every 20 a smoker, investigators report." *Washington Post*, March 24, 1915, p. 4.

11. "It's women who support cigarette industry, avers New York expert." *Washington Post*, February 7, 1916, p. 4.

12. "Miss Arnold cig. fiend." *Los Angeles Times*, March 24, 1910, p. 5.

13. Sherwood Anderson. *Winesburg, Ohio*. Mattituck, NY: Aeonian Press, 1947, pp. 148–49.

14. Allan M. Brandt. "Recruiting women smokers: the engineering of consent." *Journal of the American Medical Women's Association* (January–April, 1996): pp. 63–64.

15. "2 titled smokers." *Washington Post*, January 26, 1908, p. 13.

16. *Ibid.*

17. "Made cigarettes fashionable among women." *Los Angeles Times*, February 2, 1908, sec. 7, p. 2; "Women not to smoke," op. cit.

18. "Titled woman smokes all day." *Los Angeles Times*, April 8, 1913, p. 3.

19. "Cigars for women!" *Washington Post*, September 12, 1913, p. 6.

20. "Women not to smoke." *Washington Post*, February 9, 1908, p. E1.

21. *Ibid.*

22. "Smoking women under ban in Washington restaurants." *Washington Post*, November 13, 1911, p. 2.

23. *Ibid.*

24. "Women smoke at banquet." *Washington Post*, October 2, 1912, p. 1.

25. "Countess wants to smoke." *Washington Post*, July 7, 1909, p. 1.

26. "Woman smoked in the Ritz-Carlton." *New York Times*, December 18, 1910, p. 4.

27. "Stopped women smokers." *New York Times*, January 9, 1911, p. 1.

28. "Screens woman smoker." *Washington Post*, April 3, 1911, p. 1.

29. "Few women avail themselves of leave to whiff in hotels." *Los Angeles Times*, December 18, 1910, sec. 4, p. 11.

30. "Women may smoke there." *Washington Post*, August 26, 1910, p. 3.

31. "Cigarettes start a suffragist row." *New York Times*, September 17, 1912, p. 6.

32. "Women to smoke in hotels." *Washington Post*, September 19, 1912, p. 1.

33. "Smokes her weed in public." *Washington Post*, October 14, 1912, p. 4.

34. "Women smoke in stands." *Washington Post*, March 5, 1913, p. 18.

35. "Girl smoker invades." *Washington Post*, December 12, 1913, p. 9.

36. "Women can't smoke." *Washington Post*, April 5, 1915, p. 4.

37. "Seaside women smoke." *Washington Post*, June 22, 1915, p. 2.

38. "Baltimore women smoke at banquet for first time." *Washington Post*, February 24, 1917, p. 7.

39. "Few hotels have rules against women smokers." *New York Times Magazine*, March 16, 1919, p. 74.

40. *Ibid.*

41. "Girl arrested for smoking." *Washington Post*, May 10, 1908, p. 14.

42. "Held because she smokes." *Washington Post*, August 29, 1909, p. 13.

43. "Not crazy; brilliant." *Los Angeles Times*, September 1, 1909, p. 4.

44. "Jail woman for smoking." *Los Angeles Times*, December 16, 1912, p. 3.

45. "Cigarettes sister's bane." *New York Times*, August 18, 1909, p. 6.

46. "Woman, 61, uses cigarettes." *Washington Post*, May 24, 1913, p. 3.

47. "No more pills for Mrs. Love." *Los Angeles Times*, June 16, 1911, p. 3.

48. "Cigarettes are for all ranks." *Los Angeles Times*, January 7, 1915, sec. 2, p. 12.

49. "Court upholds women smoking." *Los Angeles Times*, March 6, 1913, p. 6.

50. "Advises smoking for women." *New York Times*, October 29, 1908, p. 12.

51. "Shall women smoke?" *Los Angeles Times*, October 31, 1908, sec. 2, p. 4.

52. "Fair smokers' mecca." *Washington Post*, April 5, 1914, p. 4.

53. "Doctor says ladies smoke." *Los Angeles Times,* July 29, 1912, p. 10.
54. "English women smoke too much." *Los Angeles Times,* May 9, 1917, sec. 2, p. 1.
55. "Girl's smoking record." *Washington Post,* September 19, 1917, p. 6.

Chapter 8

1. "Keppel raps Mrs. Longworth for smoking cigarettes." *Los Angeles Times,* August 25, 1909, p. 12.
2. "Club dames scandalized." *Los Angeles Times,* July 23, 1910, p. 7.
3. "Vote appeal to Alice." *Los Angeles Times,* August 3, 1910, p. 1.
4. "Mrs. Nick called." *Los Angeles Times,* August 5, 1910, p. 1.
5. *Ibid.*
6. "Smoking and meddling." *New York Times,* August 6, 1910, p. 6.
7. "Are the good women wise or right?" *Los Angeles Times,* August 6, 1910, sec. 2, p. 4.
8. "Mrs. Wilson against smoking by women." *New York Times,* August 13, 1912, p. 5.
9. *Ibid.*
10. "Femininity and cigarettes." *Washington Post,* January 14, 1908, p. 6.
11. "Smoking by women called deplorable." *New York Times,* January 23, 1908, p. 4.
12. "Mrs. Nation in London." *Times* (London), January 26, 1909, p. 4.
13. Lillian Bell. "Women smokers." *Washington Post,* February 18, 1909, p. 6.
14. Madison C. Peters. "The woman who smokes." *Washington Post,* December 10, 1909, p. 2.
15. "Cigarettes for Eleanor." *Los Angeles Times,* June 27, 1910, p. 11.
16. "Evils of cigarettes discussed by women." *Los Angeles Times,* June 28, 1910, p. 1.
17. "Boston bad, says pastor." *New York Times,* March 20, 1911, p. 1.
18. "Dr. Locke." *Los Angeles Times,* September 2, 1912, sec. 2, p. 3.
19. "Would cancel engagements." *Los Angeles Times,* October 3, 1912, p. 15.
20. Alma Whitaker. "Smoke screens." *Los Angeles Times,* May 15, 1927, p. L9.
21. "Smoking expensive for women." *New York Times,* February 1, 1913, p. 12.

22. Claude Cherys. "Feminine bad taste one of the crying wrongs of today." *Washington Post,* October 12, 1913, p. MT4.
23. "Blames foreign women." *Washington Post,* January 15, 1914, p. 2.
24. Eugene Brown. "Legs and cigarettes." *Los Angeles Times,* April 9, 1914, sec. 2, p. 4.
25. "Women smokers menace." *Washington Post,* December 31, 1916, p. 3.
26. Alma Whitaker. "My lady nicotine." *Los Angeles Times,* October 23, 1912, sec. 2, p. 6.
27. Alma Whitaker. "Babies and cigarettes." *Los Angeles Times,* March 21, 1916, sec. 2, p. 4.
28. Alma Whitaker. "The woman, the cigarette, the devil." *Los Angeles Times,* September 11, 1916, sec. 2, p. 4.
29. "Women smokers few." *Washington Post,* November 13, 1910, p. 11.
30. "Women fighting cigarette evil." *Los Angeles Times,* March 22, 1917, sec. 2, p. 2.
31. "Girls taboo smokers." *Washington Post,* August 1, 1911, p. 5.
32. "Clinic for women smokers." *Washington Post,* March 14, 1914, p. 1.
33. "Anti-cigarette leader in Boston on lecture tour." *Christian Science Monitor,* April 20, 1915, p. 7.
34. Frances Warfield. "Lost cause." *Outlook and Independent* 154 (February 12, 1930): 246–47.
35. "Sullivan the lesser's motion." *New York Times,* January 8, 1908, p. 8.
36. "No public smoking by women now." *New York Times,* January 21, 1908, p. 1.
37. "Women mustn't smoke." *New York Times,* January 21, 1908, p. 4.
38. "Arrested for smoking." *New York Times,* January 23, 1908, p. 1.
39. "Mayor lets women smoke." *New York Times,* February 4, 1908, p. 1.
40. "Big Tim Sullivan's idea on women cigarette smokers." *Washington Post,* February 16, 1908, pp. SM3, SM5.
41. "Tobacco-smoking females." *New York Times,* October 11, 1911, p. 1.
42. "Smoking women under ban in Washington restaurants." *Washington Post,* November 13, 1911, p. 2.
43. "A way with cigarettes." *Los Angeles Times,* January 12, 1917, sec. 2, p. 4.
44. Gordon L. Dillow. "Thank you for not smoking." *American Heritage* 32 (February/March 1981): 105.

Chapter 9

1. "War's aftermath in English cities." *New York Times*, July 11, 1920, sec. 2, p. 3.

2. "France discouraging smoking by women." *Washington Post*, August 29, 1920, p. 33.

3. "French women blamed as smoking increases." *New York Times*, August 18, 1921, p. 10.

4. "Women smokers in shops." *Times* (London), August 24, 1921, p. 5.

5. "Girl smoker wins suit." *New York Times*, January 31, 1922, p. 5.

6. "Would bar women from smoking cars." *Washington Post*, November 25, 1923, p. 19.

7. "Woman smokes before Queen at races." *New York Times*, June 19, 1924, p. 1.

8. "German bodies unite to end use of tobacco." *Washington Post*, July 20, 1924, p. ES11.

9. "Lady Astor in debate hits rum and smoking." *New York Times*, June 23, 1925, p. 13.

10. "Bryn Mawr stirs British." *New York Times*, November 25, 1925, p. 16.

11. "London smoking rooms overcrowded by women." *Washington Post*, December 7, 1926, p. 20.

12. "1,000,000 [pounds Sterling] gain in 1926 in profits on tobacco." *New York Times*, December 16, 1926, p. 45.

Chapter 10

1. "Vassar opposes women smoking." *Washington Post*, March 2, 1919, p. R2.

2. P. V. Hocking. "Campus girls puff tobacco." *Los Angeles Times*, December 19, 1920, sec. 2, p. 14.

3. "Co-eds must not smoke." *New York Times*, December 10, 1921, p. 10.

4. "Frown on smoking by co-eds in West." *New York Times*, February 14, 1922, p. 8.

5. *Ibid.*

6. "Women of West not smokers." *Los Angeles Times*, February 15, 1922, p. 6.

7. "Smoking coeds keep Nebraska teachers out of universities." *Washington Post*, February 21, 1922, p. 1.

8. "Smoking at Barnard." *New York Times*, February 26, 1922, sec. 7, p. 5.

9. *Ibid.*

10. "Michigan college sends 17 girls home." *New York Times*, April 13, 1922, p. 16.

11. "Michigan court upholds school officials." *New York Times*, March 6, 1924, p. 1.

12. Harry Burke. "Women cigarette fiends." *Ladies Home Journal* 39 (June 1922): 19.

13. "Vassar girls back anti-smoking rule." *New York Times*, November 9, 1922, p. 25.

14. "Women smokers disciplined at West Virginia University." *New York Times*, February 4, 1925, p. 23.

15. "Vassar bans smoking." *New York Times*, February 26, 1925, p. 24.

16. "M.I.T. permits smoking by women at dances." *New York Times*, October 12, 1925, p. 1.

17. "No ban at Barnard on girls' smoking." *Op. cit.*

18. "5 colleges bar girls from football dance." *New York Times*, November 19, 1925, p. 27.

19. *Ibid.*

20. "Would alter smoking plan." *New York Times*, November 20, 1925, p. 43.

21. "No ban at Barnard on girls' smoking." *New York Times*, November 25, 1925, p. 20.

22. "Bryn Mawr will allow students to smoke." *New York Times*, November 24, 1925, p. 1.

23. "Sees Bryn Mawr example." *New York Times*, November 29, 1925, p. E3.

24. "Cigarettes and college girls." *Washington Post*, November 26, 1925, p. 6.

25. "Women and the weed." *Literary Digest* 87 (December 19, 1925): 31–32.

26. "My lady nicotine gets on the campus." *New York Times Magazine*, December 27, 1925, sec. 4, p. 12.

27. "Normal school bans smoking by women." *Los Angeles Times*, December 4, 1925, p. 7.

28. "450 parents oppose smoking by girls." *New York Times*, December 20, 1925, p. 17.

29. "Club for women instructors to offer cigarettes." *Los Angeles Times*, February 1, 1926, p. 10.

30. "Smoke room for Vassar." *New York Times*, February 18, 1926, p. 6.

31. "Smoking for women." *New York Times*, March 1, 1926, p. 18.

32. "Riverside co-eds defended." *Los Angeles Times*, November 27, 1926, p. 6.

33. "Ford nurses' smoking causes an upheaval." *New York Times*, December 10, 1926, p. 3.

34. "Denies smoking story." *New York Times*, June 12, 1927, sec. 2, p. 4.

35. "Women and U.S. record of 63 billion cigarettes." *Washington Post*, January 19, 1925, p. 2.

36. Cassandra Tate. *The Triumph of the Little White Slaver*. New York: Oxford University Press, 1999, pp. 94, 106.

37. "Ask Hays to rid films of smoking by women." *New York Times*, March 1, 1922, p. 5.

38. Ernest Crutcher. "A physician's protest." *Los Angeles Times*, December 28, 1922, sec. 2, p. 6.

39. Tate, op. cit., pp. 137–38.

40. "Women smokers." *New York Times*, February 29, 1920, sec. 5, p. 9.

41. Clara Savage. "Many women secret smokers." *Washington Post*, March 13, 1921, p. 17.

42. Burke, Op cit., pp. 19, 132.

43. "Puts woman above man in morality." *New York Times*, July 20, 1924, p. 19.

44. "Why women smoke." *Washington Post*, December 17, 1924, p. 6.

45. "Why do women smoke?" *Washington Post*, October 26, 1925, p. 6.

46. "Women war-workers fight for privileges, including smoking." *Literary Digest* 61 (June 28, 1919): 76.

47. "Women's smoking room in theatre." *New York Times*, January 29, 1920, p. 9; "Smoking room for women." *New York Times*, January 9, 1922, p. 15.

48. Metcalfe. "The theatre." *Wall Street Journal*, March 19, 1923, p. 3.

49. "N.Y.A.C. permits women to smoke." *New York Times*, May 25, 1921, p. 18.

50. Helen Bullitt Lowry. "To smoke or not to smoke." *New York Times*, June 26, 1921, sec. 7, p. 9.

51. "Girl club leaders divide on smoking." *New York Times*, January 12, 1922, p. 19.

52. Burke, Op. cit., p. 19.

53. Marguerite E. Harrison. "Sorority of smoke on wheels." *New York Times Book Review and Magazine*, July 2, 1922, sec. 3, p. 2.

54. Miss Gulliver. "Smoking by the way." *New York Times Book Review and Magazine*, August 20, 1922, sec. 3, p. 11.

55. "Women invading railway smokers." *New York Times*, October 29, 1922, sec. 2, p. 5.

56. "Mixed smoking done here." *New York Times Magazine*, January 14, 1923, sec. 4, p. 2.

57. George MacAdam. "The last sanctuary of man vanishes." *New York Times*, January 4, 1925, p. SM2.

58. "Smoking bench for women." *New York Times*, July 10, 1925, p. 6.

59. "Detroit to allow women to smoke in street cars." *New York Times*, July 16, 1925, p. 1.

60. "The feminine limit." *New York Times*, July 17, 1925, p. 14.

61. "Yields on women smoking." *New York Times*, March 6, 1927, p. 2.

62. "Judge lets woman chew." *Washington Post*, September 9, 1920, p. 11.

63. "Cigarette girl held again." *New York Times*, August 7, 1922, p. 16.

64. "Enright silent about women smoking case." *New York Times*, August 20, 1922, p. 26.

65. "Extra fine for her nerve." *New York Times*, May 14, 1926, p. 9.

66. "Girl in jail a night for smoking in street." *New York Times*, July 4, 1926, p. 4.

67. "Man may ask woman for cigarette." *New York Times*, June 22, 1927, p. 29.

68. "Cigarettes blamed for whiskers." *Los Angeles Times*, August 22, 1921, p. 2; "Americans exonerate cigarette, cocktail." *Los Angeles Times*, August 23, 1921, p. 5.

69. "Women cigarette smokers." *Times* (London), September 5, 1922, p. 7.

70. Burke, op. cit.

71. Antoinette Donnelly. "Cigarettes for women." *Washington Post*, March 16, 1924, p. SM10.

72. "Women smokers." *New York Times*, November 23, 1924, sec. 9, p. 6.

73. "Doctor finds smoking ruins woman's beauty." *Washington Post*, June 7, 1925, p. E6.

74. "Women seen acquiring sallow tobacco face." *Washington Post*, January 8, 1926, p. 1.

75. "Warns against reducing." *New York Times*, March 14, 1926, p. E2.

76. "Dr. Mayo on smoking." *New York Times*, May 21, 1926, p. 22.

77. "Finds cancer a peril to women smokers." *New York Times*, May 22, 1926, p. 21.

78. "Women's voices made harsh by

smoking, specialist says." *New York Times,* August 31, 1926, p. 1.

79. Lulu Hunt Peters. "Diet and health." *Los Angeles Times,* December 29, 1926, p. A6.

Chapter 11

1. "Nicotine next." *Times* (London), August 7, 1919, p. 10.

2. "Women are smoking more." *Washington Post,* February 6, 1920, p. 6.

3. "Sensation menaced by smoking women." *New York Times,* February 6, 1920, p. 13.

4. "Women smokers." *New York Times,* February 29, 1920, sec. 5, p. 9.

5. "Bar women's cigarettes." *New York Times,* June 24, 1920, p. 6.

6. "Smoking will continue." *New York Times,* June 25, 1920, p. 11

7. "Dr. Wise denounces lipstick and wine." *New York Times,* March 21, 1921, p. 12

8. "Grandmamma's cigarette." *New York Times,* April 21, 1921, p. 12.

9. "Let girls smoke, Mrs. Du Puy's plea." *New York Times,* October 15, 1921, p. 8.

10. "National council bans cigarettes for women." *New York Times,* November 16, 1921, p. 10.

11. "Frown on women smokers." *New York Times,* January 29, 1922, sec. 2, p. 2.

12. "Girls ban jazz, petting parties, cigarettes." *New York Times,* February 18, 1922, p. 4.

13. "War on smoking among women." *Los Angeles Times,* May 6, 1922, p. 3.

14. "Greenwich Village stirs judge's ire." *New York Times,* May 12, 1922, p. 8.

15. "Tobacco state's governor would aid women's clubs to put ban on cigarettes." *New York Times,* January 30, 1924, p. 21.

16. Mildred Holland. "Making the most of personality." *Washington Post,* March 18, 1924, p. 10.

17. Leslie S. Reed. "Burbank urges fight on weed." *Los Angeles Times,* July 20, 1924, p. B24.

18. "Fiske tells girls to stop smoking." *New York Times,* November 20, 1924, p. 21.

19. "Bars smoking on graves." *New York Times,* September 17, 1925, p. 25.

20. "Anti-tobacconists in the United States." *Times* (London), October 20, 1925, tobacco supp., p. 30.

21. E. D. Goode. "Tobacco habit." *Los Angeles Times,* December 7, 1925, p. A4.

22. "Mrs. Henderson, hostess, leads dress reform fight." *Washington Post,* December 27, 1925, p. 1.

23. "Society women hit at immodest dress." *New York Times,* December 27, 1925, p. 14.

24. "Women in villages held more moral than society girls." *Washington Post,* December 28, 1925, p. 2.

25. Alma Whitaker. "Very smokey." *Los Angeles Times,* January 10, 1926, p. L7.

26. "Tobacco men to unite to fight the W.C.T.U." *New York Times,* October 10, 1919, p. 18.

27. "Seeking no law to ban tobacco." *New York Times,* November 13, 1919, sec. 2, p. 2.

28. "Women smokers." *New York Times,* February 29, 1920, sec. 5, p. 9.

29. "Antitobacco movement on." *Los Angeles Times,* April 4, 1921, p. 6.

30. "Café smoking hit by women." *Los Angeles Times,* April 20, 1923, sec. 2, pp. 1–2.

31. "To bar women smokers." *New York Times,* March 17, 1925, p. 24.

32. "Try to censure Queen on smoking." *New York Times,* October 22, 1926, p. 8.

33. Jacob Sullum. *For Your Own Good: The Anti-Smoking Crusade and the Tyranny of Public Health.* New York: Free Press, 1998, p. 37.

34. Frances Warfield. "Lost cause." *Outlook and Independent* 154 (February 12, 1930): 247.

35. *Ibid.,* p. 275.

36. "Cigarette plea to Harding." *New York Times,* December 20, 1920, p. 3.

37. "Cigarettes for Harding." *New York Times,* December 23, 1920, p. 3; "Send cigarettes to Harding; prosecution is demanded." *New York Times,* December 24, 1960, p. 1.

38. "Harding thinks tobacco foes should not be hypocrites." *New York Times,* January 17, 1921, p. 15.

39. "Cigarette foe dismissed." *New York Times,* January 24, 1921, p. 5.

40. "Finds kick in cigarette." *New York Times,* January 25, 1922, p. 19.

41. "Evils laid to cigarettes." *Los Angeles Times,* November 17, 1923, sec. 2, pp. 1, 6.

42. Warfield, op. cit., pp. 275–76.
43. "Would ban public smoking by women." *Washington Post*, June 21, 1921, p. 10.
44. "Bill to stop women smoking in Washington." *New York Times*, June 21, 1921, p. 1.
45. "Crime in Washington." *New York Times*, June 22, 1921, p. 14.
46. Helen Bullitt Lowry. "To smoke or not to smoke." *New York Times*, June 26, 1921, sec. 7, p. 2.
47. *Ibid.*
48. "Saving our women." *Los Angeles Times*, July 22, 1921, sec. 2, p. 4.
49. "Women of Washington to fight ban on smoking." *New York Times*, July 28, 1921, p. 1.
50. "To curb women smokers." *New York Times*, March 7, 1922, p. 30.
51. "A cause worth attention." *New York Times*, March 8, 1922, p. 14.
52. "Seeks to stop women smoking in the open." *New York Times*, December 21, 1921, p. 11.
53. "Smoking in public barred for women; police enforce law." *New York Times*, March 28, 1922, p. 1.
54. *Ibid.*, p. 4.
55. Raymond C. Carroll. "No smoking rule big joke on city." *Washington Post*, March 29, 1922, p. 5.
56. "Licenses to live, die, eat or think, urged." *Washington Post*, March 30, 1922, p. 11.
57. "Votes to end Kansas cigarette ban." *New York Times*, February 25, 1925; "Ends anti-cigarette law." *New York Times*, February 4, 1927, p. 6.

smoker." *New York Times*, July 9, 1930, p. 24.
6. "Smoking in higher places." *New York Times*, July 10, 1930, p. 24.
7. "Women cause Reich railroads to give half train to smokers." *New York Times*, May 19, 1929, p. E3.
8. "Nazi women bar cosmetics." *New York Times*, August 11, 1933, p. 10; "Reich tightens curb on Jewish doctors." *New York Times*, August 20, 1933, p. 5; "Curb on smoking widened." *New York Times*, September 17, 1933, p. 12.
9. "Reich's women smokers warned on motherhood." *New York Times*, August 23, 1937, p. 7.
10. "Germany bans free beer and tobacco for workers." *New York Times*, May 13, 1939, p. 2.
11. "Germany bans smoking by girls at universities." *New York Times*, June 8, 1940, p. 3.
12. "Nazis cut cigarettes to 3 daily." *New York Times*, January 21, 1942, p. 7.
13. "Britons hear plea to curtail smoking." *New York Times*, July 7, 1941, p. 4.
14. "French women propose they get cigarettes too." *New York Times*, November 19, 1944, p. 8; "Frenchwomen thwarted in cigarette ration trick." *New York Times*, March 1, 1945, p. 18.
15. "French minister refuses tobacco cards to women." *New York Times*, July 20, 1945, p. 7.
16. "Women's tobacco ration is approved in France." *New York Times*, September 14, 1945, p. 14.
17. "British women go for gaspers." *Washington Post*, May 18, 1958, p. E5.

Chapter 12

1. "Women smoke for France." *New York Times*, February 5, 1928, sec. 9, p. 4.
2. "Women smokers hit by French devotees." *New York Times*, November 19, 1928, p. 2.
3. "Few Frenchwomen are real smokers." *Washington Post*, September 13, 1934, p. 15.
4. "Cocoa trust's demise laid to girl smokers." *New York Times*, August 30, 1928, p. 30.
5. "Queen Mary pictured as regular

Chapter 13

1. "College dean bans smoking by women." *Christian Science Monitor*, November 7, 1929, p. 1.
2. "Smoking co-eds penalized." *New York Times*, March 15, 1930, p. 10.
3. "Smoking to cost girls diplomas." *Los Angeles Times*, February 14, 1931, p. A1.
4. "Smoking just women's fad, says college head." *Los Angeles Times*, March 30, 1933, p. A2.
5. "Lady nicotine triumphs in Fresno

co-eds' vote." *Los Angeles Times*, October 13, 1933, p. 9.

6. "Smoking co-eds." *Literary Digest* 123 (May 15, 1937): 28.

7. *Ibid.*

8. "Smoking history and background." Online Document,www.webspawner.com/users/smokingbackground, January 2004.

9. "Women can now smoke in Marine Corps offices." *Washington Post*, July 22, 1927, p. 20.

10. "Cigarette sales in America gain 90 percent in seven years by aid of women." *Los Angeles Times*, August 9, 1927, p. 11.

11. "Woman no longer hides her cigarette." *New York Times Magazine*, August 28, 1927, sec. 4, p. 19.

12. Alma Whitaker. "Her cigarette." *Los Angeles Times*, April 14, 1929, p. G15.

13. *Ibid.*

14. "Lady smokers blacklisted." *Los Angeles Times*, February 16, 1930, p. 2.

15. "The smokier sex." *New York Times*, May 7, 1930, p. 26.

16. "Rural areas frown on women smokers." *New York Times*, September 19, 1931, p. 19.

17. "Women and cigarettes." *Printers' Ink* 158 (February 18, 1932): 25.

18. *Ibid.*, pp. 25, 27.

19. *Ibid.*, p. 27.

20. Virginia L. Ernster. "Mixed messages for women." *New York State Journal of Medicine* 85 (July 1985): 337.

21. "Smoking rule works one way." *Los Angeles Times*, November 29, 1934, p. 4.

22. "Mrs. Luce urges smoking cut." *New York Times*, December 2, 1944, p. 15.

23. George Gallup. "52 per cent of civilians smoke." *Los Angeles Times*, December 22, 1944, p. 7.

24. "Cigarette producers seeking sales of 400 billion annually." *New York Times*, March 11, 1946, p. 32.

25. "Smoke pressure." *Christian Science Monitor*, March 21, 1946, p. 22.

26. George Gallup. "Poll upholds smoking by women teachers." *Los Angeles Times*, November 23, 1946, p. 1.

27. George Gallup. "Cigarettes smoked by 44 percent in poll." *Los Angeles Times*, December 19, 1949, p. 20.

28. "Survey finds U.S. has 38 million smokers." *Washington Post*, June 22, 1955, p. 21.

29. "Tobacco." *Time* 75 (April 11, 1960): 104.

30. "Hotel's ban on smoking irks women." *Los Angeles Times*, July 29, 1927, p. 2.

31. "See hails club ban on smoking by women." *New York Times*, August 30, 1927, p. 1.

32. "Automatic cigarette machines." *Wall Street Journal*, September 14, 1928, p. 5.

33. "M'Elligott pleads to ban store smoking." *New York Times*, December 12, 1936, p. 8.

34. "30-year ban on smoking is lifted at Bedford." *New York Times*, December 25, 1933, p. 34.

35. "Woman no longer hides her cigarette." *New York Times Magazine*, August 28, 1927, sec. 4, p. 19.

36. Edward L. Bernays. *Biography of an Idea: Memoirs of Public Relations Counsel Edward L. Bernays*. New York: Simon and Schuster, 1965, pp. 386–87.

37. "Easter Sun." *New York Times*, April 1, 1929, pp. 1, 3.

38. "Smoking of women on streets is upheld." *Washington Post*, July 14, 1931, p. 12.

39. "Town riled by woman smoking pipe in public." *Washington Post*, August 31, 1934, p. 12.

40. "Topics of the Times." *New York Times*, June 28, 1949, p. 26.

41. "Babies held poisoned by smoking mothers." *Washington Post*, September 24, 1927, p. 3.

42. "Doctors deny smoking mothers poison babes." *Washington Post*, September 25, 1927, p. M7.

43. "Those cigaret-smoking mothers." *Hygeia* 5 (November 1927): 583.

44. "Smoking mothers." *Scientific American* 152 (April 1935): 217–18.

45. William L. Laurence. "Headaches eased with vitamin B." *New York Times*, June 12, 1942, p. 23.

46. William Brady. "Here's to health." *Los Angeles Times*, June 12, 1944, p. A10.

47. "Says smoking robs women of beauty." *New York Times*, October 10, 1928, p. 30.

48. "Fags blamed for women's facial droop." *Los Angeles Times*, August 17, 1931, p. 1.

49. Allan L. Benson. "Smokes for women." *Good Housekeeping* 89 (August 1929): 190–91.

50. *Ibid.*, pp. 192–93.

51. Lydia Lane. "Beauty rules tobacco's use." *Los Angeles Times*, January 30, 1935, p. A5.

52. "Smoking called coronary heart disease factor." *Los Angeles Times*, March 27, 1948, p. 1.

53. "Denies cancer threat to women who smoke." *New York Times*, May 16, 1928, p. 8.

54. "Physician says smoking may cause lung cancer." *Los Angeles Times*, January 23, 1953, p. 21.

55. "Mayor of Lynn bars movies which show girls smoking." *New York Times*, October 17, 1929, p. 1.

56. "New film ban proposed." *Los Angeles Times*, April 10, 1930, pp. A1–A2.

57. "Bill hits at women smoking on screen." *Los Angeles Times*, January 20, 1933, p. 3; "Hays ethics code evaded by trickery." *Los Angeles Times*, March 5, 1933, p. A1.

58. "Films blamed by W.C.T.U. for women's cigarettes." *Los Angeles Times*, August 9, 1938, p. 6.

59. "Smoking history and background," op. cit.; Ernster, op. cit., p. 337.

60. Eunice Fuller Barnard. "The cigarette has made its way up in society." *New York Times*, June 9, 1929, p. SM18.

61. Allan M. Brandt. "Recruiting women smokers: the engineering of consent." *Journal of the American Medical Women's Association* (January–April 1996): 64.

62. Ernster, op. cit., p. 336.

63. "Blow some more my way." *Printers' Ink* 159 (April 14, 1932): 20.

64. "Cigarette sales in America gain 90 percent in seven years by aid of women." *Los Angeles Times*, August 9, 1927, p. 11.

65. Ernster, op. cit.

66. Richard Kluger. *Ashes to Ashes*. New York: Alfred A. Knopf, 1996, p. 74.

67. Louis Proyect. "Women and cigarettes." Online Document, http://csf.colorado.edu, January 2004.

68. Alma Whitaker. "Her cigarette." *Los Angeles Times*, April 14, 1929, p. G15.

69. "Diva denies addiction to smoking." *Los Angeles Times*, February 13, 1927, p. 3.

70. "Two women testify at FTC hearing here." *New York Times*, April 5, 1944, p. 30.

71. "Albert Lasker." Online Document, www.ciadvertising.org, January 2004.

72. Brandt, op. cit., pp. 64–65.

73. *Ibid.*, pp. 65–66.

74. "Cigarette concern stops health ads." *New York Times*, January 24, 1930, p. 20.

75. Virginia L. Ernster, op. cit., p. 337.

76. "Fight launched on radio boosts for cigarette use." *Los Angeles Times*, December 10, 1928, p. 4.

77. F. M. Gregg. "Insidious cigarette advertising protested by college professor." *Christian Science Monitor* (May 2, 1929): 6.

78. *Ibid.*

79. "Fag billboards drawing fire." *Los Angeles Times*, May 8, 1929, p. 12.

80. "Club women frown on cigarette ads." *Christian Science Monitor*, May 21, 1929, p. 2.

81. Ernster, op. cit., p. 336.

82. "The cigarette evil." *Christian Science Monitor*, September 21, 1929, p. 22.

83. "Methodists assail tobacco concerns." *Washington Post*, December 6, 1929, p. 5.

84. "Seeks check by law on cigarette ads." *New York Times*, February 3, 1930, p. 9.

Chapter 14

1. "Women smokers leading the nation to ruin." *New York Times*, July 8, 1927, p. 2.

2. "Booking of preacher canceled." *Los Angeles Times*, January 2, 1928, p. 7.

3. "Sex equality in smoking urged." *Los Angeles Times*, January 9, 1928, p. 4.

4. "Women, religion and cigarets." *Literary Digest* 96 (January 28, 1928): 28–29.

5. *Ibid.*

6. "Maude Royden's cigarets." *Literary Digest* 96 (February 4, 1928): 32.

7. "Tobacco smoke clouds issue." *Los Angeles Times*, February 24, 1928, p. A10.

8. "Dr. Wilson attacks cigarette campaign of tobacco trust." *Washington Post*, May 6, 1929, p. 16.

9. "Church fights home wine." *Los Angeles Times*, February 16, 1931, p. 1.

10. "Pastor belittles dry law killings." *New York Times*, April 8, 1929, p. 21.

11. "Modern girls hit by Catholic youth." *Washington Post*, July 14, 1929, p. M3.

12. "Catholic heads oppose smoking among women." *Los Angeles Times*, June 23, 1931, p. 2.

13. "Scouts will combat smoking by women." *Washington Post*, July 7, 1928, p. 1.

14. "Breakers just ahead." *New York Times*, July 9, 1928, p. 18.

15. "Boy Scout body bans drive on girls' smoking." *New York Times*, July 13, 1928, p. 19.

16. Allan L. Benson. "Smokes for women." *Good Housekeeping* 89 (August 1929): 40.

17. "Forming league to oppose women and minors smoking." *New York Times*, December 9, 1930, p. 22.

18. "Town code for teachers bars women who smoke." *New York Times*, September 9, 1933, p. 15.

19. "Women's styles and manners as- sailed by Mrs. Richardson." *Washington Post*, March 19, 1935, p. 14.

20. "Public smoking a vicious habit." *Washington Post*, October 22, 1937, p. 3.

21. "Gelett Burgess in your life." *Reader's Digest* 33 (July 1938): 68.

22. "Smoking's bad for everyone, says Teamster chief Tobin." *Los Angeles Times*, April 9, 1950, p. 13.

Bibliography

"Advanced woman upheld." *New York Times*, September 2, 1895, p. 5.
"Advises smoking for women." *New York Times*, October 29, 1908, p. 12.
"Advises women to smoke." *New York Times*, August 27, 1906, p. 1.
"Albert Lasker." Online Document, www.ciadvertising.org, January 2004.
"American tobacco is pushed abroad." *New York Times*, July 28, 1929, sec. 3, p. 7.
"Americans exonerate cigarette, cocktail." *Los Angeles Times*, August 23, 1921, p. 5.
Anderson, Sherwood. *Winesburg, Ohio*. Mattituck, NY: Aeonian Press, 1947.
"Anti-cigarette leader in Boston on lecture tour." *Christian Science Monitor* (April 20, 1915): 7.
"Antitobacco movement on." *Los Angeles Times*, April 4, 1921, p. 6.
"Anti-tobacconists in the United States." *Times* (London), October 20, 1925, tobacco supp., p. 30.
Apperson, G. L. *The Social History of Smoking*. London: Martin Secker, 1914.
"Are the good women wise or right?" *Los Angeles Times*, August 6, 1910, sec. 2, p. 4.
"Arrested for smoking." *New York Times*, January 23, 1908, p. 1.
"Ask Hays to rid films of smoking by women." *New York Times*, March 1, 1922, p. 5.
"Assert women are smokers." *Los Angeles Times*, October 28, 1912, p. 3.
"Automatic cigarette machines." *Wall Street Journal*, September 14, 1928, p. 5.
"Babies held poisoned by smoking mothers." *Washington Post*, September 24, 1927, p. 3.
"Baltimore women smoke at banquet for first time." *Washington Post*, February 24, 1917, p. 7.
Banks, Elizabeth. "English women smoke cigarettes." *Washington Post*, October 26, 1902, p. 19.
"Bar women's cigarettes." *New York Times*, June 24, 1920, p. 6.
Barnard, Eunice Fuller. "The cigarette has made its way up in society." *New York Times*, June 9, 1929, pp. SM6, SM8.
"Bars bridge and smoking." *New York Times*, July 23, 1907, p. 4.
"Bars smoking on graves." *New York Times*, September 17, 1925, p. 25.
Barton, Alexander. "Should women smoke?" *Washington Post*, October 2, 1904, p. B3.
Bell, Lillian. "Women smokers." *Washington Post*, February 18, 1909, p. 6.
Benson, Allan L. "Smokes for women." *Good Housekeeping* 89 (August 1929): 190–94.
Bernays, Edward L. *Biography of an Idea: Memoirs of Public Relations Counsel Edward L. Bernays*. New York: Simon and Schuster, 1965.
Biddle, Elizabeth. "Cigarette smoking among Englishwomen no uncommon practice." *New York Times*, March 25, 1906, p. SM7.
"Big Tim Sullivan's ideas on women cigarette smokers." *Washington Post*, February 16, 1908, pp. SM3, SM5.
"Bill hits at women smoking on screen." *Los Angeles Times*, January 20, 1933, p. 3.
"Bill to stop women smoking in Washington." *New York Times*, June 21, 1921, p. 1.
"Blames foreign women." *Washington Post*, January 15, 1914, p. 2.

"Blow some more my way." *Printers' Ink* 159 (April 14, 1932): 20.

"Booking of preacher canceled." *Los Angeles Times*, January 2, 1928, p. 7.

"Boston bad, says pastor." *New York Times*, March 20, 1911, p. 1.

"Boy Scout body bans drive on girls' smoking." *New York Times*, July 13, 1928, p. 19.

Brady, William. "Here's to health." *Los Angeles Times*, June 12, 1944, p. A10.

Brandt, Allan M. "Recruiting women smokers: the engineering of consent." *Journal of the American Medical Women's Association* (January-April 1996): 63–66.

"Breakers just ahead." *New York Times*, July 9, 1928, p. 18.

"British women go for gaspers." *Washington Post*, May 18, 1958, p. E5.

"Britons hear plea to curtail smoking." *New York Times*, July 7, 1941, p. 4.

Brown, Eugene. "Legs and cigarettes." *Los Angeles Times*, April 9, 1914, sec. 2, p. 4.

"Bryn Mawr stirs British." *New York Times*, November 25, 1925, p. 16.

"Bryn Mawr will allow students to smoke." *New York Times*, November 24, 1925, p. 1.

Burke, Harry. "Women cigarette fiends." *Ladies Home Journal* 39 (June 1922): 19, 132.

"Café smoking hit by women." *Los Angeles Times*, April 20, 1923, sec. 2, pp. 1–2.

Carroll, Raymond G. "No smoking rule big joke on city." *Washington Post*, March 29, 1922, p. 5.

"Catholic heads oppose smoking among women." *Los Angeles Times*, June 23, 1931, p. 2.

"A cause worth attention." *New York Times*, March 8, 1922, p. 14.

Cherys, Claude. "Feminine bad taste one of the crying wrongs of today." *Washington Post*, October 12, 1913, p. MT4.

"Church fights home wine." *Los Angeles Times*, February 16, 1931, p. 1.

"Cigarette concern stops health ads." *New York Times*, January 24, 1930, p. 20.

"The cigarette evil." *Christian Science Monitor*, September 21, 1929, p. 22.

"Cigarette foe dismissed." *New York Times*, January 24, 1921, p. 5.

"Cigarette girl held again." *New York Times*, August 7, 1922, p. 16.

"Cigarette habit grips women." *Los Angeles Times*, September 22, 1907, sec. 7, p. 6.

"Cigarette habit growing among Washington women?" *Washington Post*, April 1, 1906, p. E6.

"The cigarette hoarders." *Weekly Dispatch* (UK), December 9, 1917, p. 3.

"Cigarette plea to Harding." *New York Times*, December 20, 1920, p. 3.

"Cigarette producers seeking sales of 400 billion annually." *New York Times*, March 11, 1946, p. 32.

"Cigarette sales in America gain 90 percent in seven years by aid of women." *Los Angeles Times*, August 9, 1927, p. 11.

"Cigarette-smoking women." *Washington Post*, February 1, 1891, p. 4.

"Cigarettes and college girls." *Washington Post*, November 26, 1925, p. 6.

"Cigarettes and fair fingers." *Washington Post*, February 16, 1896, p. 22.

"Cigarettes are for all ranks." *Los Angeles Times*, January 7, 1915, sec. 2, p. 12.

"Cigarettes blamed for whiskers." *Los Angeles Times*, August 22, 1921, p. 2.

"Cigarettes fashionable?" *Los Angeles Times*, April 19, 1906, sec. 2, p. 13.

"Cigarettes for Eleanor." *Los Angeles Times*, June 27, 1910, p. 11.

"Cigarettes for Harding." *New York Times*, December 23, 1920, p. 3.

"Cigarettes sister's bane." *New York Times*, August 18, 1909, p. 6.

"Cigarettes start a suffragist row." *New York Times*, September 17, 1912, p. 6.

"Cigars for women!" *Washington Post*, September 12, 1913, p. 6.

"Clinic for women smokers." *Washington Post*, March 14, 1914, p. 1.

"Club dames scandalized." *Los Angeles Times*, July 23, 1910, p. 2.

"Club for women instructors to offer cigarettes." *Los Angeles Times*, February 1, 1926, p. 10.

"Club women frown on cigarette ads." *Christian Science Monitor*, May 21, 1929, p. 2.

"Cocoa trust's demise laid to girl smokers." *New York Times*, August 30, 1928, p. 30.

"Co-eds must not smoke." *New York Times*, December 10, 1921, p. 10.

"College dean bans smoking by women." *Christian Science Monitor*, November 7, 1929, p. 1.

"Countess wants to smoke." *Washington Post*, July 7, 1909, p. 1.

"Court upholds women smoking." *Los Angeles Times*, March 6, 1913, p. 6.
"Crime in Washington." *New York Times*, June 22, 1921, p. 14.
Crutcher, Ernest. "A physician's protest." *Los Angeles Times*, December 28, 1922, sec. 2, p. 6.
"Curb on smoking widened." *New York Times*, September 17, 1933, p. 12.
"Czarina forbids smoking." *Los Angeles Times*, February 18, 1908, sec. 2, p. 4.
"Dainty cigarettes for women." *Washington Post*, December 15, 1895, p. 20.
"Delmonico bars women smokers." *Los Angeles Times*, October 22, 1897, p. 14.
"Denies cancer threat to women who smoke." *New York Times*, May 16, 1928, p. 8.
"Denies smoking story." *New York Times*, June 12, 1927, sec. 2, p. 4.
"Detroit to allow women to smoke in street cars." *New York Times*, July 16, 1925, p. 1.
"Die then, and smoke, said his majesty." *Los Angeles Times*, June 28, 1901, p. 1.
Dillow, Gordon L. "Thank you for not smoking." *American Heritage* 32 (February/March 1981): 94–107.
"Disobeying Queen Mary." *Los Angeles Times*, May 14, 1911, pp. 1–2.
"Diva denies addiction to smoking." *Los Angeles Times*, February 13, 1927, p. 3.
"Doctor finds smoking ruins woman's beauty." *Washington Post*, June 7, 1925, p. E6.
"Doctor says ladies smoke." *Los Angeles Times*, July 29, 1912, p. 10.
"Doctors deny smoking mothers poison babes." *Washington Post*, September 25, 1927, p. M7.
Donnelly, Antoinette. "Cigarettes for women." *Washington Post*, March 16, 1924, p. SM10.
"Dr. Locke." *Los Angeles Times*, September 2, 1912, sec. 2, p. 3.
"Dr. Mayo on smoking." *New York Times*, May 21, 1926, p. 22.
"Dr. Wilson attacks cigarette campaign of tobacco trust." *Washington Post*, May 6, 1929, p. 16.
"Dr. Wise denounces lipstick and wine." *New York Times*, March 21, 1921, p. 12.
"Duchess smokes cigars." *Washington Post*, December 21, 1913, p. 1.
Dunhill, Alfred. "The woman's pipe." *Times* (London), October 20, 1925, tobacco supp., p. 21.
"Easter Sun." *New York Times*, April 1, 1929, pp. 1, 3.
"Ends anti-cigarette law." *New York Times*, February 4, 1927, p. 6.
"English women smoke too much." *Los Angeles Times*, May 9, 1917, sec. 2, p. 1.
"Enright silent about woman smoking case." *New York Times*, August 20, 1922, p. 26.
Ernster, Virginia L. "Mixed messages for women." *New York State Journal of Medicine* 85 (July 1985): 335–40.
"Evils laid to cigarettes." *Los Angeles Times*, November 17, 1923, sec 2, pp. 1, 6.
"Evils of cigarettes discussed by women." *Los Angeles Times*, June 28, 1910, p. 1.
"Extra fine for her nerve." *New York Times*, May 14, 1926, p. 9.
"Fag billboards drawing fire." *Los Angeles Times*, May 8, 1929, p. 12.
"Fags blamed for women's facial droop." *Los Angeles Times*, August 17, 1931, p. 1.
"Fair smokers' mecca." *Washington Post*, April 5, 1914, p. 4.
"Fashion's frivolities." *Weekly Dispatch* (UK), February 25, 1900, p. 15.
"The feminine limit." *New York Times*, July 17, 1925, p. 14.
"Feminine smokers." *Washington Post*, March 2, 1890, p. 15.
"Femininity and cigarettes." *Washington Post*, January 14, 1908, p. 6.
"Few Frenchwomen are real smokers." *Washington Post*, September 13, 1934, p. 15.
"Few hotels have rules against women smokers." *New York Times Magazine*, March 16, 1919, p. 74.
"Few women avail themselves of leave to whiff in hotels." *Los Angeles Times*, December 18, 1910, sec. 4, p. 11.
"The field is the world." *New York Times*, February 13, 1919, p. 14.
"Fight launched on radio boosts for cigarette use." *Los Angeles Times*, December 10, 1928, p. 4.
"Films blamed by W.C.T.U. for women's cigarettes." *Los Angeles Times*, August 9, 1938, p. 6.
"Finds cancer a peril to women smokers." *New York Times*, May 22, 1926, p. 21.

"Finds kick in cigarette." *New York Times*, January 25, 1922, p. 19.

"Fiske tells girls to stop smoking." *New York Times*, November 20, 1924, p. 21.

"5 colleges bar girls from football dance." *New York Times*, November 19, 1925, p. 27.

"Ford nurses' smoking causes an upheaval." *New York Times*, December 10, 1926, p. 3.

"Forming league to oppose women and minors smoking." *New York Times*, December 9, 1930, p. 22.

"450 parents oppose smoking by girls." *New York Times*, December 20, 1925, p. 17.

"France discouraging smoking by women." *Washington Post*, August 29, 1920, p. 33.

"French minister refuses tobacco cards to women." *New York Times*, July 20, 1945, p. 7.

"French women blamed as smoking increases." *New York Times*, August 18, 1921, p. 10.

"French women propose they get cigarettes too." *New York Times*, November 19, 1944, p. 8.

"Frenchwomen thwarted in cigarette ration trick." *New York Times*, March 1, 1945, p. 18.

"From snuff to cigarettes." *Washington Post*, March 26, 1906, p. 6.

"Frown on smoking by co-eds in West." *New York Times*, February 14, 1922, p. 8.

"Frown on women smokers." *New York Times*, January 29, 1922, sec. 2, p. 2.

Gallup, George. "Cigarettes smoked by 44% in poll." *Los Angeles Times*, December 19, 1949, p. 20.

Gallup, George. "52 per cent of civilians smoke." *Los Angeles Times*, December 22, 1944, p. 7.

Gallup, George. "Poll upholds smoking by women teachers." *Los Angeles Times*, November 23, 1946, p. 1.

"Gelett Burgess in your life." *Reader's Digest* 33 (July 1938): 68.

"German bodies unite to end use of tobacco." *Washington Post*, July 20, 1924, p. ES11.

"Germany bans free beer and tobacco for workers." *New York Times*, May 13, 1939, p. 2.

"Germany bans smoking by girls at university." *New York Times*, June 8, 1940, p. 3.

"Girl arrested for smoking." *Washington Post*, May 10, 1908, p. 14.

"Girl club leaders divide on smoking." *New York Times*, January 12, 1922, p. 19.

"Girl in jail a night for smoking in street." *New York Times*, July 4, 1926, p. 4.

"Girl smoker invades." *Washington Post*, December 12, 1913, p. 9.

"Girl smoker wins suit." *New York Times*, January 31, 1922, p. 5.

"Girls ban jazz, petting parties, cigarettes." *New York Times*, February 18, 1922, p. 4.

"Girl's smoking record." *Washington Post*, September 19, 1917, p. 6.

"Girls taboo smokers." *Washington Post*, August 1, 1911, p. 5.

Goode, E. D. "Tobacco habit." *Los Angeles Times*, December 7, 1925, p. A4.

"Grandmamma's cigarette." *New York Times*, April 21, 1921, p. 12.

"Greenwich Village stirs judge's ire." *New York Times*, May 12, 1922, p. 8.

Gregg, F. M. "Insidious cigarette advertising protested by college professor." *Christian Science Monitor*, May 2, 1929, pp. 1, 6.

Gulliver, Miss. "Smoking by the way." *New York Times Book Review and Magazine*, August 20, 1922, sec. 3, p. 11.

"Harding thinks tobacco foes should not be hypocrites." *New York Times*, January 17, 1921, p. 15.

Harrison, Marguerite E. "Sorority of smoke on wheels." *New York Times Book Review and Magazine*, July 2, 1922, sec. 3, p. 2.

Hawthorne, Julian. "Can ladies smoke tobacco?" *Washington Post*, October 25, 1903, p. F3.

"Hays ethics code evaded by trickery." *Los Angeles Times*, March 5, 1933, p. A1.

"Held because she smokes." *Washington Post*, August 29, 1909, p. 13.

"The history of tobacco, part II (1700–1899)." History Net. Online Document, www.historian.org, January 2004.

Hocking, P. V. "Campus girls puff tobacco." *Los Angeles Times*, December 19, 1920, sec. 2, p. 14.

Holland, Mildred. "Making the most of personality." *Washington Post*, March 18, 1924, p. 10.

"Hotel's ban on smoking irks women." *Los Angeles Times*, July 29, 1927, p. 2.

"It's women who support cigarette industry, avers New York expert." *Washington Post*, February 7, 1916, p. 4.

"Jail woman for smoking." *Los Angeles Times*, December 16, 1912, p. 3.

"Judge lets woman chew." *Washington Post*, September 9, 1920, p. 11.

"Keppel raps Mrs. Longworth for smoking cigarettes." *Los Angeles Times*, August 25, 1909, p. 12.

"King's ransom goes in smoke." *Los Angeles Times*, December 19, 1914, sec. 2, pp. 1, 6.

Kluger, Richard. *Ashes to Ashes*. New York: Alfred A. Knopf, 1996.

"Lady Astor in debate hits rum and smoking." *New York Times*, June 23, 1925, p. 13.

"Lady nicotine triumphs in Fresno co-eds' vote." *Los Angeles Times*, October 13, 1933, p. 9.

"Lady smokers blacklisted." *Los Angeles Times*, February 16, 1930, p. 2.

"Lady smokers of England." *Los Angeles Times*, July 8, 1906, sec. 1, p. 6.

Lander, Meta. *The Tobacco Problem* 6th ed. 1882; Boston: Lee and Shepard, 1899.

Lane, Lydia. "Beauty rules tobacco's use." *Los Angeles Times*, January 30, 1935, p. A5.

Laurence, William L. "Headaches eased with vitamin B." *New York Times*, June 12, 1942, p. 23.

"Let girls smoke, Mrs. Du Puy's plea." *New York Times*, October 15, 1921, p. 8.

"Licenses to live, die, eat or think urged." *Washington Post*, March 30, 1922, p. 11.

"London smoking rooms overcrowded by women." *Washington Post*, December 7, 1926, p. 20.

"London women smoke in public." *Los Angeles Times*, November 26, 1899, p. 30.

"London's women smokers." *Washington Post*, February 23, 1902, p. 34.

Lowry, Helen Bullitt. "To smoke or not to smoke." *Los Angeles Times*, June 26, 1921, sec. 7, pp. 2, 9.

MacAdam, George. "The last sanctuary of man vanishes." *New York Times*, January 4, 1925, p. SM2.

"Made cigarettes fashionable among women." *Los Angeles Times*, February 2, 1908, sec. 7, p. 2.

"Man may ask woman for cigarette." *New York Times*, June 22, 1927, p. 29.

"Many women are smokers." *Los Angeles Times*, January 5, 1908, sec. 1, p. 4.

"Maude Royden's cigarets." *Literary Digest* 96 (February 4, 1928): 32.

"May women smoke in auto?" *New York Times*, September 26, 1904, p. 1.

"Mayor lets women smoke." *New York Times*, February 4, 1908, p. 1.

"Mayor of Lynn bans movies which show girls smoking." *New York Times*, October 17, 1929, p. 1.

"M'Elligott pleads to ban store smoking." *New York Times*, December 12, 1936, p. 8.

Metcalfe. "The theatre." *Wall Street Journal*, March 19, 1923, p. 3.

"Methodists assail tobacco concerns." *Washington Post*, December 6, 1929, p. 5.

M'Guirk, Mrs. "Lady cigarettes." *Los Angeles Times*, March 18, 1894, p. 15.

"Michigan college sends 17 girls home." *New York Times*, April 13, 1922, p. 16.

"Michigan court upholds school officials." *New York Times*, March 6, 1924, p. 1.

"Milady puffs cigars." *Washington Post*, March 22, 1914, p. 2.

"Miss Arnold cig. fiend." *Los Angeles Times*, March 24, 1910, p. 5.

"Miss Gaston begins anti-cigarette war." *New York Times*, September 12, 1907, p. 2.

"M.I.T. permits smoking by women at dances." *New York Times*, October 12, 1925, p. 1.

"Mixed smoking done here." *New York Times Magazine*, January 14, 1923, sec. 4, p. 2.

"Modern girls hit by Catholic youth." *Washington Post*, July 14, 1929, p. M3.

"Mrs. Henderson, hostess, leads dress reform fight." *Washington Post*, December 27, 1925, pp. 1, 16.

"Mrs. Luce urges smoking cut." *New York Times*, December 2, 1944, p. 15.

"Mrs. Nation in London." *Times* (London), January 26, 1909, p. 4.

"Mrs. Nick called." *Los Angeles Times*, August 5, 1910, p. 1.

"Mrs. Wilson against smoking by women." *New York Times*, August 13, 1912, p. 5.

"My lady nicotine gets on the campus." *New York Times Magazine*, December 27, 1925, sec. 4, pp. 12, 22.

"National council bans cigarettes for women." *New York Times*, November 16, 1921, p. 10.

"Nazi women bar cosmetics." *New York Times*, August 11, 1933, p. 10.

"Nazis cut cigarettes to three daily." *New York Times*, January 21, 1942, p. 7.

"New film ban proposed." *Los Angeles Times*, April 10, 1930, pp. A1–A2.

"Newport to war on smoking by women." *New York Times*, May 3, 1908, p. 11.

"Nicotine next." *Times* (London), August 7, 1919, p. 10.

"No ban at Barnard on girls' smoking." *New York Times*, November 25, 1925, p. 20.

"No more pills for Mrs. Love." *Los Angeles Times*, June 16, 1911, p. 3.

"No public smoking by women now." *New York Times*, January 21, 1908, p. 1.

"Normal school bans smoking by women." *Los Angeles Times*, December 4, 1925, p. 7.

"Not all may smoke." *Washington Post*, January 5, 1908, p. 10.

"Not crazy; brilliant." *Los Angeles Times*, September 1, 1909, p. 4.

"N.Y.A.C. permits women to smoke." *New York Times*, May 25, 1921, p. 18.

"Objects to women smoking." *New York Times*, January 11, 1913, p. 1.

"1,000,000 [pounds Sterling] gain in 1926 in profits on tobacco." *New York Times*, December 16, 1926, p. 45.

"One woman in Chicago of every 20 a smoker, investigators report." *Washington Post*, March 24, 1915, p. 4.

"Online exhibits: Carry A. Nation." Kansas State Historical Society, Online Document, www.kshs.org, January 2004.

"Pastor belittles dry law killings." *New York Times*, April 8, 1929, p. 21.

Peters, Lulu Hunt. "Diet and health." *Los Angeles Times*, December 29, 1926, p. A6.

Peters, Madison C. "The woman who smokes." *Washington Post*, December 10, 1909, p. 2.

"Physician says smoking may cause lung cancer." *Los Angeles Times*, January 23, 1953, p. 21.

Proyect, Louis. "Women and cigarettes." Online Document, http://csf.colorado.edu, January 2004.

"Public smoking a vicious habit." *Washington Post*, October 22, 1937, p. 3.

"Puffs rings of smoke while taking the air." *Los Angeles Times*, December 7, 1912, p. 1.

"Puts woman above man in morality." *New York Times*, July 20, 1924, p. 19.

"Queen Mary pictured as regular smoker." *New York Times*, July 9, 1930, p. 9.

Reed, Leslie S. "Burbank urges fight on weed." *Los Angeles Times*, July 20, 1924, p. B24.

"Reich tightens curb on Jewish doctors." *New York Times*, August 20, 1933, p. 5.

"Reich's women smokers warned on motherhood." *New York Times*, August 23, 1937, p. 7.

"Riverside co-eds defended." *Los Angeles Times*, November 27, 1926, p. 6.

Rudy, Jarrett. "Unmaking manly smokers: church, state, governance, and the first anti-smoking campaigns in Montreal, 1892–1914." *Journal of the Canadian Historical Association* 12 (2001): 95–114.

"Rural areas frown on women smokers." *New York Times*, September 19, 1931, p. 19.

Ryan, Marion. "All the men and women merely wills's." *Weekly Dispatch* (UK), November 25, 1917, p. 4.

Savage, Clara. "Many women secret smokers." *Washington Post*, March 13, 1921, p. 17.

"Saving our women." *Los Angeles Times*, July 22, 1921, sec. 2, p. 4.

"Says smoking robs women of beauty." *New York Times*, October 10, 1928, p. 30.

"Scoff at W.C.T.U." *Washington Post*, August 21, 1910, p. 9.

"Scouts will combat smoking by women." *Washington Post*, July 7, 1928, p. 1.

"Screens woman smoker." *Washington Post*, April 3, 1911, p. 1.

"Seaside women smoke." *Washington Post*, June 22, 1915, p. 2.

"See hails club ban on smoking by women." *New York Times*, August 30, 1927, p. 21.

"Seeking no law to bar tobacco." *New York Times*, November 13, 1919, sec. 2, p. 2.

"Seeks check by law on cigarette ads." *New York Times*, February 3, 1930, p. 9.

"Seeks to stop women smoking in the open." *New York Times*, December 21, 1921, p. 11.

"Sees Bryn Mawr example" *New York Times*, November 29, 1925, p. E3.

"Send cigarettes to Harding; prosecution is demanded." *New York Times*, December 24, 1920, p. 1.

"Sensation menaced by smoking women." *New York Times*, February 6, 1920, p. 13.
"Sex equality in smoking urged." *Los Angeles Times*, January 9, 1928, p. 4.
"Shall women smoke?" *Los Angeles Times*, November 13, 1893, p. 4.
"Shall women smoke?" *Los Angeles Times*, October 31, 1908, sec. 2, p. 4.
"She smoked on the Avenue." *Washington Post*, December 29, 1895, p. 2.
"Should women smoke?" *Washington Post*, March 6, 1892, p. 12.
"Smoke pressure." *Christian Science Monitor*, March 21, 1946, p. 22.
"Smoke room for Vassar." *New York Times*, February 18, 1926, p. 6.
"Smoked 1907 out." *Washington Post*, January 1, 1908, p. 1.
"Smokers among the fair sex." *Washington Post*, February 28, 1904, p. A8.
"Smokes her weed in public." *Washington Post*, October 14, 1912, p. 4.
"The smokier sex." *New York Times*, May 7, 1930, p. 26.
"Smoking among women." *Washington Post*, July 30, 1911, p. E4.
"Smoking and meddling." *New York Times*, August 6, 1910, p. 6.
"Smoking at Barnard." *New York Times*, February 26, 1922, sec. 7, p. 5.
"Smoking bench for women." *New York Times*, July 10, 1925, p. 6.
"Smoking by women called deplorable." *New York Times*, January 23, 1908, p. 4.
"Smoking called coronary heart disease factor." *Los Angeles Times*, March 27, 1948, p. 1.
"Smoking car for women?" *New York Times*, March 22, 1906, p. 1.
"Smoking co-eds." *Literary Digest* 123 (May 15, 1937): 28.
"Smoking co-eds keep Nebraska teachers out of universities." *Washington Post*, February 21, 1922, p. 1.
"Smoking co-eds penalized." *New York Times*, March 15, 1930, p. 10.
"Smoking expensive for women." *New York Times*, February 1, 1913, p. 12.
"Smoking for women." *New York Times*, March 1, 1926, p. 18.
"Smoking history and background." Online Document,www.webspawner.com/users/smokingbackground, January 2004.
"Smoking in high places." *New York Times*, July 10, 1930, p. 24.
"Smoking in public barred for women; police enforce law." *New York Times*, March 28, 1922, pp. 1, 4.
"Smoking just women's fad, says college head." *Los Angeles Times*, March 30, 1933, p. A2.
"Smoking mothers." *Scientific American* 152 (April 1935): 217–18.
"Smoking of women on streets is upheld." *Washington Post*, July 14, 1931, p. 12.
"Smoking on increase here." *Washington Post*, December 19, 1912, p. 4.
"Smoking: online exhibits." Kansas State Historical Society, Online Document, www.kshs.org, January 2004.
"Smoking room for women." *New York Times*, January 9, 1922, p. 15.
"Smoking rule works one way." *Los Angeles Times*, November 29, 1934, p. 4.
"Smoking to cost girls diplomas." *Los Angeles Times*, February 14, 1931, p. A1.
"Smoking will continue." *New York Times*, June 25, 1920, p. 11.
"Smoking women augment." *New York Times*, March 6, 1898, p. 7.
"Smoking women under ban in Washington restaurants." *Washington Post*, November 13, 1911, p. 2.
"Smoking's bad for everyone, says Teamster chief Tobin." *Los Angeles Times*, April 9, 1950, p. 13.
"Society women hit at immodest dress." *New York Times*, December 27, 1925, p. 14.
"Society women smoking." *Washington Post*, July 16, 1893, p. 12.
"Society's new woman." *Washington Post*, June 2, 1895, p. 14.
"Stop smoking them, boys." *Washington Post*, November 24, 1890, p. 8.
"Stopped women smokers." *New York Times*, January 9, 1911, p. 1.
Studholme, Marie. "Should women smoke?" *Washington Post*, October 2, 1904, p. B3.
"Sullivan the lesser's motion." *New York Times*, January 8, 1908, p. 8.
Sullum, Jacob. *For Your Own Good: The Anti-Smoking Crusade and the Tyranny of Public Health.* New York: Free Press, 1998.

"Survey finds U.S. has 38 million smokers." *Washington Post*, June 22, 1955, p. 21.
Tate, Cassandra. *The Triumph of the Little White Slaver*. New York: Oxford University Press, 1999.
"30-year ban on smoking is lifted at Bedford." *New York Times*, December 25, 1933, p. 34.
"Those cigaret-smoking mothers." *Hygeia* 5 (November 1927): 583.
"Tiny pipes for women." *Washington Post*, July 8, 1888, p. 12.
"Titled woman smokes all day." *Los Angeles Times*, April 8, 1913, p. 3.
"To bar women smokers." *New York Times*, March 17, 1925, p. 24.
"To curb women smokers." *New York Times*, March 7, 1922, p. 30.
"To reform Paris also." *New York Times*, June 21, 1908, p. C2.
"Tobacco." *Time* 75 (April 11, 1960): 104–6.
"Tobacco men unite to fight the W.C.T.U." *New York Times*, October 10, 1919, p. 18.
"Tobacco smoke clouds issue." *Los Angeles Times*, February 24, 1928, p. A10.
"Tobacco-smoking females." *New York Times*, October 11, 1911, p. 1.
"Tobacco state's governor would aid women's clubs to put ban on cigarettes." *New York Times*, January 20, 1924, p. 21.
"Topics of the Times." *New York Times*, June 28, 1949, p. 26.
"Town code for teachers bans women who smoke." *New York Times*, September 9, 1933, p. 15.
"Town riled by woman smoking pipe in public." *Washington Post*, August 31, 1934, p. 12.
Troyer, Ronald J. and Gerald E. Markle. *Cigarettes: The Battle over Smoking*. New Brunswick, NJ: Rutgers University Press, 1983.
"Try to censure Queen on smoking." *New York Times*, October 22, 1926, p. 8.
"2 titled smokers." *Washington Post*, January 26, 1908, pp. 1, 13.
"Two women testify at FTC hearing here." *New York Times*, April 5, 1944, p. 30.
"Under W.C.T.U. ban." *New York Times*, May 18, 1907, p. 6.
"Use of cigarettes." *Los Angeles Times*, April 1, 1897, p. 8.
"Use of snuff increasing." *Los Angeles Times*, February 11, 1899, p. 7.
"The use of tobacco." *New York Times*, September 14, 1874, p. 3.
"Varieties." *News of the World* (UK), June 20, 1886, p. 6.
"Vassar bans smoking." *New York Times*, February 26, 1925, p. 24.
"Vassar girls back anti-smoking rule." *New York Times*, November 9, 1922, p. 25.
"Vassar opposed women smoking." *Washington Post*, March 2, 1919, p. R2.
"The Victorian days." *Times* (London), December 30, 1926, p. 6.
"The Victorian days." *Times* (London), January 1, 1927, p. 6.
"The Victorian days." *Times* (London), January 3, 1927, p. 8.
"The Victorian days." *Times* (London), January 4, 1927, p. 6.
"Vote appeal to Alice." *Los Angeles Times*, August 3, 1910, p. 1.
"Votes to end Kansas cigarette ban." *New York Times*, February 25, 1925, p. 20.
"War on smoking among women." *Los Angeles Times*, May 6, 1927, p. 3.
Warfield, Frances. "Lost cause." *Outlook and Independent* 154 (February 12, 1930): 244–47, 275–76.
"Warns against reducing." *New York Times*, March 14, 1926, p. E2.
"War's aftermath in English cities." *New York Times*, July 11, 1920, sec. 2, p. 3.
"A way with cigarettes." *Los Angeles Times*, January 12, 1917, sec. 2, p. 4.
"Where a woman shares man's joy in pipe and cigar." *Washington Post*, July 30, 1905, p. B5.
Whitaker, Alma. "Babies and cigarettes." *Los Angeles Times*, March 21, 1916, sec. 2, p. 4.
Whitaker, Alma. "Her cigarette." *Los Angeles Times*, April 14, 1929, p. G15.
Whitaker, Alma. "My lady nicotine." *Los Angeles Times*, October 23, 1912, sec. 2, p. 6.
Whitaker, Alma. "Smoke screens." *Los Angeles Times*, May 15, 1927, p. L9.
Whitaker, Alma. "The woman, the cigarette, the devil." *Los Angeles Times*, September 11, 1916, Sec. 2, p. 4.
Whitaker, Alma. "Very smokey." *Los Angeles Times*, January 10, 1926, p. L7.
"Why do women smoke?" *Washington Post*, October 26, 1925, p. 6.

"Why women smoke." *Washington Post*, December 17, 1924, p. 6.
"Will the coming woman smoke?" *Los Angeles Times*, August 20, 1893, p. 12.
"Woman and home." *Los Angeles Times*, March 30, 1893, p. 10.
"Woman no longer hides her cigarette." *New York Times Magazine*, August 28, 1927, sec. 4, p. 19.
"Woman, 61, uses cigarettes." *Washington Post*, May 24, 1913, p. 3.
"Woman smoked in the Ritz-Carlton." *New York Times*, December 18, 1910, p. 4.
"Woman smokers before Queen at races." *New York Times*, June 19, 1924, p. 1.
"Woman with tobacco heart." *Los Angeles Times*, March 7, 1907, sec. 1, p. 14.
"Women abuse the weed." *New York Times*, May 21, 1913, p. 3.
"Women aid U.S. record of 63 billion cigarettes." *Washington Post*, January 19, 1925, p. 2.
"Women and cigarettes." *Washington Post*, December 30, 1895, p. 6.
"Women and cigarettes." *Washington Post*, March 29, 1906, p. A1.
"Women and cigarettes." *Printers' Ink* 158 (February 18, 1932): 25–27.
"Women and smoking." *New York Times*, September 1, 1879, p. 2.
"Women and the weed." *Literary Digest* 87 (December 19, 1925): 31–32.
"Women and tobacco." *New York Times*, February 28, 1897, p. SM5.
"Women are smoking now." *Washington Post*, February 6, 1920, p. 6.
"Women can't smoke." *Washington Post*, April 5, 1915, p. 4.
"Women cause Reich railroads to give half train to smokers." *New York Times*, May 19, 1929, p. E3.
"Women cigarette smokers." *New York Times*, June 24, 1901, p. 7.
"Women cigarette smokers." *Times* (London), September 5, 1922, p. 7.
"Women fighting cigarette evil." *Los Angeles Times*, March 22, 1917, sec. 2, p. 2.
"Women in villages held more moral than society girls." *Washington Post*, December 28, 1925, p. 2.
"Women invading railway smokers." *New York Times*, October 29, 1922, sec. 2, p. 5.
"Women may smoke there." *Washington Post*, August 26, 1910, p. 3.
"Women mustn't smoke." *New York Times*, January 22, 1908, p. 4.
"Women not to smoke." *Washington Post*, February 9, 1908, p. E1.
"Women now can smoke in Marine Corps offices." *Washington Post*, July 22, 1927, p. 20.
"Women of Washington fight ban on smoking." *New York Times*, July 28, 1921, p. 1.
"Women of West not smokers." *Los Angeles Times*, February 15, 1922, p. 6.
"Women, religion, and cigarets." *Literary Digest* 96 (January 28, 1928): 28–29.
"Women seen acquiring sallow tobacco face." *Washington Post*, January 8, 1926, p. 1.
"Women smoke at banquet." *Washington Post*, October 2, 1912, p. 1.
"Women smoke for France." *New York Times*, February 5, 1928, sec. 9, p. 4.
"Women smoke in stands." *Washington Post*, March 5, 1913, p. 18.
"Women smoke less." *Washington Post*, November 29, 1908, p. 17.
"Women smokers." *New York Times*, February 29, 1920, sec. 5, p. 9.
"Women smokers." *New York Times*, November 23, 1924, sec. 9, p. 6.
"Women smokers disciplined at West Virginia University." *New York Times*, February 4, 1925, p. 23.
"Women smokers few." *Washington Post*, November 13, 1910, p. 11.
"Women smokers hit by French devotees." *New York Times*, November 19, 1928, p. 2.
"Women smokers in shops." *Times* (London), August 24, 1921, p. 5.
"Women smokers leading the nation to ruin." *New York Times*, July 8, 1927, p. 2.
"Women smokers menace." *Washington Post*, December 31, 1916, p. 3.
"Women to smoke in hotels." *Washington Post*, September 19, 1912, p. 1.
"Women using narcotics." *New York Times*, January 10, 1897, p. 13.
"Women war-workers fight for privileges, including smoking." *Literary Digest* 61 (June 28, 1919): 76.
"Women who smoke." *Washington Post*, November 4, 1888, p. 9.
"Women who smoke." *Washington Post*, November 25, 1888, p. 12.

"The women who smoke." *New York Times*, December 3, 1907, p. 8.

"Women who smoke rare." *New York Times*, December 9, 1894, p. 18.

"Women's cigarette holders." *Los Angeles Times*, December 8, 1912, sec. 3, p. 25.

"Women's smoking room in theatre." *New York Times*, January 29, 1920, p. 9.

"Women's styles and manners assailed by Mrs. Richardson." *Washington Post*, March 19, 1935, p 14.

"Women's tobacco ration is approved in France." *New York Times*, September 14, 1945, p. 14.

"Women's voices made harsh by smoking, specialist says." *New York Times*, August 31, 1926, p. 1.

"Would alter smoking plan." *New York Times*, November 20, 1925, p. 43.

"Would ban public smoking by women." *Washington Post*, June 21, 1921, p. 10.

"Would bar women from smoking cars." *Washington Post*, November 25, 1923, p. 19.

"Would cancel engagements." *Los Angeles Times*, October 3, 1912, p. 15.

"Would tar Stotesbury." *Washington Post*, January 13, 1913, p. 1.

"Yields on women smoking." *New York Times*, March 6, 1927, p. 2.

Index

239

Washington University 156
weight loss 129, 186, 192–195
Wellesley College 101–102, 105–106
Wessel, Curtis A. 163
West, James E. 208
West Virginia University 104
Whitaker, Alma 52–53, 85, 87–88, 138, 159–160, 186–187
White, Maude 74
Wichita 38
Williams, Milton B. 40
Williamson, O. 184
wills contested 75
Wilson, Clarence True 201, 206–207
Wilson, Ellen 80–81

Wise, Stephen S. 133
Woman's Christian Temperance Union (WCTU) 40–45, 79, 88, 138–141
woman's place 36–37
Woodbury, Levi 66
Woodward, Cora Stranahan 61
Wooten, Harry W. 164–165
World War I 10, 55–57, 76–77
World War II 154–155
wrappers, cigarette 9

Yawger, Frances 132
YMCA 10
YWCA 57, 65; British 57